Closing the Pleasure Gap

Closing the Pleasure Gap

An Ob-Gyn Explains What Women Want in Bed

Dr Amrinder Bajaj

HAY HOUSE

HAY HOUSE INDIA
New Delhi • London • Sydney
Carlsbad, California • New York City

Hay House Publishers (India) Pvt Ltd
Muskaan Complex, Plot No. 3, B-2, Vasant Kunj, New Delhi – 110070, India

Hay House LLC, P.O. Box 5100, Carlsbad, CA 92018-5100, USA
Hay House UK Ltd, 1st Floor, Crawford Corner, 91-93 Baker Street, London W1U 6QQ, UK
Hay House Australia Publishing Pty Ltd, 18/36 Ralph St., Alexandria NSW 2015, Australia

Email: contact@hayhouse.co.in
Website: www.hayhouse.co.in

First published by Hay House India, 2026
10 9 8 7 6 5 4 3 2 1

ISBN 978-93-6611-481-1 (Paperback)
ISBN 978-93-6611-025-7 (Ebook)

Printed at Thomson Press India Private Limited

FSC www.fsc.org MIX Paper | Supporting responsible forestry FSC® C010615

Hay House is committed to a sustainable future for our business, our readers and our planet. This book is made from Forest Stewardship Council® certified paper.

for
my unfulfilled sisters

Contents

Foreword

The title of this book, *Closing the Pleasure Gap: An Ob-Gyn Explains What Women Want in Bed*, may appear titillating to some. But I can assure them that this is a scholarly work on a serious subject of the utmost importance for men and women. Especially men. Dr Amrinder Bajaj is eminently qualified to write it. She is a highly qualified doctor and a gold medallist who specialised in Obstetrics and Gynaecology from AIIMS. She was formerly head of the Department of Obstetrics and Gynaecology at Max Hospital, Pitampura, and an educator at Medicity Gurgaon, and is at present a Senior Consultant at Fortis Memorial Research Institute (FMRI).

The subject is important because of the pervasive ignorance among those who think they know all about it. The degree of ignorance in both men and women about sex appears to be in inverse proportion to their obsession with it. Men who claim to be great lovers are usually the most ignorant. They know a great deal about how to please themselves, but not half as much as they should about how to please those who are the source of that pleasure: Women.

This may seem odd when never before in the history of mankind has there been so much public prominence and social sanction accorded to the practice and projection of sex. Sex is everywhere: On billboards, on television, in newspapers and magazines, in books and films, and in the vast domain of cyberspace. The problem lies, perhaps, precisely in this surfeit. There is so much about sex in our daily existence that we have forgotten what true and fulfilling sensuality is.

In the Hindu worldview, the four highest *purusharthas*, or goals of life, are *Dharma*, *Artha*, *Kama*, and *Moksha*. The sage

Vatsyayana, who almost two thousand years ago wrote the *Kama Sutra*, states that if the first three of these goals—Dharma (right conduct), Artha (the acquisition of material well-being), and Kama (the pursuit of desire)—are followed in proportion as part of a balanced life, then Moksha, or salvation, the fourth and final goal, is the natural consequence.

In other words, in the Hindu approach, Kama, or sensual emotion, was never denigrated. On the contrary, Kama has a place among the four highest goals of life, and in religion, Kama is also considered a most powerful deity. If, therefore, Kama is one of the most important goals of life, then it is not enough, Vatsyayana argues, to be merely any kind of lover. One must be an accomplished lover. A man who merely uses a woman for an uncontrollably brief moment of physical friction, giving unilateral satisfaction to himself, is undesirable—even uncultured—and almost a catastrophe for many women who have finally begun to discover their sensuality and want the optimum from sex.

I find it nothing short of amazing that Indian civilisation was possibly the first in the world to articulate the theory, as the *Kama Sutra* does, that men must respect the sensuality of women, realise that women can differ in their expectations of good sex, have different needs, and be equal partners in sensual pleasure. In fact, Vatsyayana exhorts a man to do what a woman enjoys, to interpret her needs, and to understand her preferences. The keyword here is 'respect'.

But this respect cannot be given until men are educated and women become aware of their own potential. This is why Dr Amrinder Bajaj's book is a must-read for both sexes. With empathy and deep knowledge, she elucidates what a woman wants in bed, the ways for her to achieve fulfilment, how important it is for her to know her own anatomy and psyche, and, above all, how imperative it is for men to know how to please her.

There are also many other aspects of sex on which Dr Bajaj writes with clarity and depth. Such effortless and clinical fluency can only come to a person who, for decades as a top-notch practising doctor, has been a careful and sympathetic observer of the prevailing ignorance on a subject which, otherwise, should be a source, between consenting adults and husband and wife, of immense and mutual pleasure.

I would like to congratulate her on a necessary, timely, and impeccably researched book. In Indian civilisation, *avidya*, or ignorance, is considered the root cause of delusion, pain, and suffering. Dr Bajaj has undertaken the task of providing vidya on a subject that is very much a pivotal part of the lives of men and women. The book, while universal in its message, is especially relevant to Indians where—thanks to centuries of gender discrimination and subordination—most men are sensually insensitive and women sexually deprived.

—Pavan K. Varma
Author, former Member of Parliament at the Rajya Sabha, and former diplomat

***The sexual revolution has been great—
for men.***

Our ancestors believed that good sex ensured a stable marriage; a stable marriage ensured a stable society; and a stable society sustained a stable kingdom.

To illustrate this belief, there is an apocryphal story from the thirteenth century, set in an eastern kingdom of India. A king was seated with his ministers when a naked woman ran into the court. The scandalised ministers rushed forward to clothe her, but she stopped them.

'I am fed up,' she said. 'I have always taken care to fully pleasure all my lovers, yet no man has ever taken the trouble to satisfy me completely. I have decided that, until a man is able to satisfy me fully, I will not dress again.'

The men panicked at the prospect of this becoming the norm, imagining their own women taking to the streets naked if dissatisfied in bed. Realising that the stability of his kingdom was at stake, the king asked whether any man present believed himself capable of satisfying her. One man came forward and was, apparently, successful, for the woman returned to court the following day fully clothed.

Author's Note

Forty-five years ago, Polish gynaecologist Michalina Wisłocka put in a great effort to get her book on female sexuality published. She was called a slut, a madwoman, amongst other names, but she persevered against overwhelming odds.

When her book, *The Art of Loving*, was finally released in 1978, it went on to sell seven million copies. This shows how starved women were of sexual knowledge—from a woman's perspective.

Women in modern-day India, the land of the *Kama Sutra*, fare no better than their Polish counterparts. And who should know better than me, a gynaecologist privy to their innermost secrets? It saddens me to state that a vast number of women have never experienced the supreme pleasure their bodies can give them. Barring a few, most men are either ignorant of or indifferent to a woman's needs in bed. It is time that the other half of the world's population got its due.

Whatever explicit content there is in this book is derived from treatises on sex written by our ancients. I marvel at the time and effort they invested, the passion with which they indulged in the most pleasurable of activities known to man, unlike the perpetual hurry of present-day living in all matters, especially those that matter most.

A proverb by Sheikh Nefzaoui, the fifteenth-century author of *The Perfumed Garden*, describes it best: 'A humid kiss is better than a hurried coitus.'

Our very own Sage Vatsyayana, author of the *Kama Sutra*, stated two thousand years ago that men and women are equal partners in the act of consummation, and the fulfilment of a woman is at the heart of the experience of sex.

What happened to these teachings? Were the prudish Mughal and British invaders to blame? Did they shame and suppress the most enjoyable part of a man–woman relationship?

Even in this so-called modern age, girls are brought up to feel ashamed of their private parts. They are told that virginity is a treasure that must be guarded with their lives. After marriage, she submits to the advances of a stranger who ravishes her without finesse or concern, scarring her for life. No matter how distasteful the act, she has to accommodate her husband, for men have special 'needs'. Those who develop a taste for sex as a recreational activity end up feeling guilty for such shameful propensities, as society would like to pretend that female sexuality does not exist, though '*sambhog*' a Hindi word for intercouse, means 'equal pleasure'.

The poetess Forugh Farrokhzad was the first woman to openly declare the existence of female sexuality in conservative Iran of the fifties; she paid a heavy price for it. The lines below in her famous poem 'Sin' are about rebellion, not remorse—a challenge to society and religion, not an expression of guilt:

> I sinned a sin full of pleasure,
> In an embrace which was warm and fiery.
> I sinned surrounded by arms
> that were hot and avenging and iron.

Cultures that acknowledge its existence curb it with chastity belts in ancient times or with female genital mutilation, which is prevalent even today.

What is it that men fear? That, given free rein, their women would run amok? Or is it due to a deep-rooted insecurity that stems from the fact that, while a woman is 100 per cent sure that she is the mother of the child she gives birth to, a man—before DNA testing became available—could never be certain that the child he was raising was his? Since prehistoric times, he would drag a woman by her hair to his cave to ensure that the child she bore was his. The bangles, anklets, and nose pins we wear with such pleasure are not mere ornaments, but vestiges of shackles, manacles, and nose rings once used by men to restrain women and ensure paternity.

Paradoxically, he will go to bizarre extremes to procure the prohibited tiger claw or rhino horn to increase his prowess. Why? So that he can impregnate as many women as possible and carry his genes forward. Instead of depleting wildlife to extinction, all he has to do is treat her like a person and play upon her beautiful body like a flute, till she opens up to him like a flower and explodes in ecstasy. It is time the world realised that orgasm is the right of every woman.

Sad to say, even the medical profession lags in addressing female sexuality and the management of FSD (female sexual disorders). According to Charles Runels, MD, 'men and their doctors have significantly more options to help with sexual function than do women and their clinicians. Moreover, the education of physicians regarding the examination and treatment of women for sexual dysfunction has been—and remains, even in 2024—much less thorough than for men.'[1] Drugs for the management of FSDs are far fewer than the plethora of remedies available for men with sexual dysfunction.

Around the time the book and film *Fifty Shades of Grey* were released, *Newsweek* put it on its cover. At an airport, Dr Runels bought the magazine, showed it to the woman sitting next to him, and asked, 'What do you think—is this the new' sexual revolution?'

She replied, 'In the '60s, it became okay for women to have sex; now, it's okay for women to demand good sex.' He wanted to add, '. . . and they want to define for themselves what 'good' means.'

Yet sex is not all about ecstasy. There are consequences one must keep in mind before indulging in bodily pleasures. The couple—more so the woman—should be aware of the fallout of irresponsible sexual behaviour, for she has to bear the brunt of such activities. This could range from unwanted pregnancies and illegal abortions to sexually transmitted infections, chronic inflammation of the genital tract leading to blocked tubes and infertility, not to mention pain during intercourse that ruins her sex life and drives her partner to seek solace elsewhere. Like my Polish counterpart, I have seen the havoc wrought on the female body and psyche by poor or non-existent sex education.

As Asif Becher stated in his review of the film *The Art of Loving* (on Michalina Wisłocka's life and times), she had seen in Poland 'women dying of botched, illegal abortions, marriages torn apart by infidelity and dissatisfaction, and a country full of miserable people who can't seem to find a way to talk about something they all do.' This is what I see in India today.

⚤

The objective of this book is to create a society that embraces female sexuality without belittling it—a culture that gives her the pleasure it expects to receive from her, treats her as a person to be loved and respected, not as an object to be used or abused. I do not intend to declare war between the two sexes, for nothing can be more beautiful than a relationship wherein both partners complete each other, like the halves of a whole. One's pleasure can only be enhanced by pleasuring the other. A man who understands a woman's needs and satisfies her as he would like his own needs to be satisfied is blessed, for he will reap its benefits a hundred times over.

A soaring of passions, like powerful winged birds,
a cataract of pleasure cascading over flesh,
grim determined pursuits without civilised graces.
The grappling and groping as if battling for life,
like two wild animals in lethal combat.
Faces curiously contorted, as if in pain.
The exquisite torture, the tormenting clasp,
the building of pressures, the straining, the striving,
the rapturous convulsions, the shuddering release,
the uncoiling of tension, the languorous stupor.
A bounty greater than this can nature bestow?

Part I

Female Sexuality

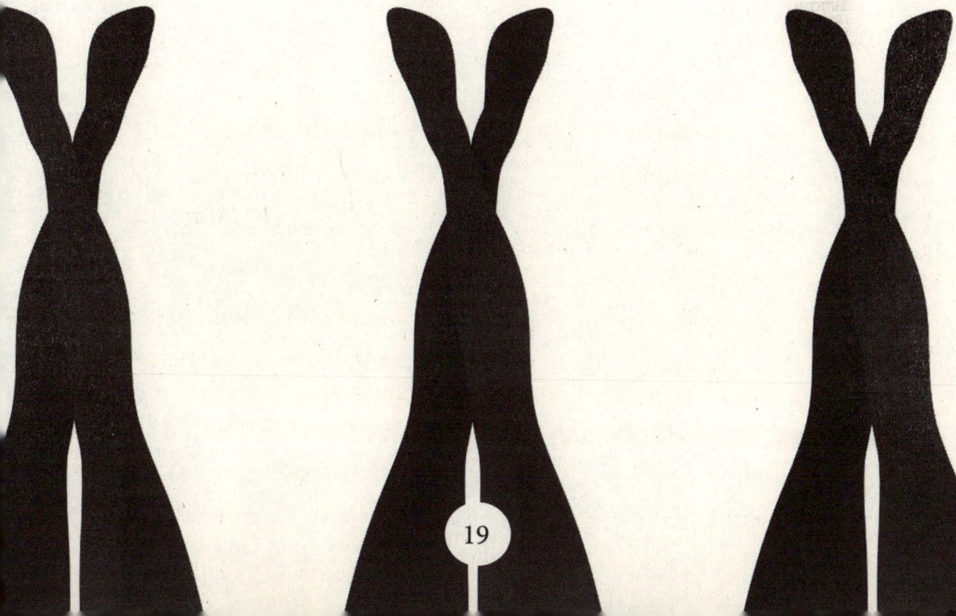

1

Society and the Female Sex

I was often reprimanded by my parents, as a girl, for questioning their double standards. My brothers could swim and stay out late; I was not allowed to do so. I was scolded for raising my voice because, in my time, girls were brought up to become spineless, voiceless dolls, trained to function as subservient slaves in their *sasurals*.

Years later, I submitted meekly to an arranged marriage, though I was repulsed by the idea. By then, I had become culturally conditioned to comply, as generations of Indian girls had done before me. As for attempting to equate my status with that of my brothers, my mother pronounced with a finality that brooked no argument: 'Girls get pregnant; boys do not.'

She was right. As a gynaecologist, I encounter unmarried girls who suffer the consequences of clandestine abortions. What troubled me, however, was the absence of an equal emphasis on teaching sons not to indiscriminately impregnate vulnerable women.

Our mindset is such that girls who wear Western clothes are labelled hot and sexy, while those who dress conservatively are dismissed as *behenjis*. A girl who is friendly with boys is branded a slut; a boy who sleeps around is celebrated as a stud. More often than not, women are objectified—*cheez*, *maal*, *pataka*—not to mention slurs that reduce her to her sex organs. To many men, she is chiefly about breasts, genitalia, and availability. Even our swear words are directed at women. That she is an intelligent, affectionate human being, capable of offering far more than her body, does not register.

Women in the West fare no better, judging by the steady stream of sex scandals emerging from Hollywood. There, too, jokes about dumb blondes abound, while blonde men escape scrutiny.

Superwomen that we are, we toil at home and outside it; we manage children, demanding in-laws, guests in the dining room, and a husband in bed—often without appreciation or support. At times, the husband seeks the services of a mistress to satisfy his 'needs', which an exhausted and depleted housewife may be unable to fulfil.

Certain questions about gender inequality continue to trouble me:

- Why is it important for a girl to enter the bridal chamber with her hymen intact, while virginity is not a precondition for her groom? I am not advocating promiscuity, merely exposing the double standards entrenched in our society.
- Why is the raped woman victimised, and not the rapist?
- Why does the husband's family demand dowry when it is *streedhan*—the wealth a father gives his daughter, from ancient times, in lieu of the property he bestows upon his sons? It belongs solely to her, to use freely or retain as a safety net in dire circumstances.
- Why do women endure domestic violence, as though they deserve it?
- Why is a woman labelled *banj* (barren) in an infertile marriage, when the fault—if it is a fault at all—may lie with the man?
- Why is she blamed for producing daughters, when the 'Y' chromosome required for a male child comes from the husband?
- Why does she risk her life aborting female foetuses until she proves her worth as the mother of a son?
- And, last but not least, why does she tolerate all this?

Perhaps it is to preserve her 'married' status, for she is socially, financially, emotionally, and sexually dependent on her husband. Even women who are financially independent often remain trapped in toxic marriages—some even handing over their salaries to their lord and master—out of fear of ostracism or of living alone in a predatory world. The mantle of a 'married' woman offers protection in a society that views divorcees, widows, and single women as easy prey. Many are denied refuge in their parental homes, for *'sasural se ladki ki arthi nikalti hai'*. More often than not, this grim prophecy is fulfilled through in-laws who burn her alive when their demands are unmet. I am ashamed to say that the term 'dowry death' is peculiar to my country, India. Parents, too, bear responsibility when they turn their daughters away when she needs them most.

We can put an end to this rampant victimisation of women by celebrating the birth of a daughter as joyously as that of a son; by offering equal love, nutrition, education, and opportunity to both; by teaching sons to treat women with respect; by making women aware of their rights and instilling in them the courage to defend those rights; and, finally, by enforcing zero tolerance for sexist behaviour in the workplace.

We are guaranteed equality under the Constitution. So, why do we permit ourselves to be treated as second-class citizens? It is a proven fact that women are the stronger sex in matters that truly matter. Why, then, do we not draw upon our collective strength to improve our lot?

In the bargain of life, it's our lot to give,
and yet be grateful for being allowed to live,
for the female foetus is killed before birth
and the girl child simply fades from earth.
As mother, mistress, wife, and maid,
solely to serve her man she's made.
From acid attacks, stalking, and rape,
how do these hapless victims escape?

Many a Gayatri, Gunjan, Gauri
have been sacrificed for dowry.
Nutrition for childbearing *she* needs,
yet the best portions, to her man she feeds.
A barren woman they quickly replace
for many are waiting to take her place.
If daughters are all that she can deliver,
shamed, she hides to cower and quiver.
Each breath is beholden to his breath,
for a widow's life is worse than death.
What amazes is the acceptance of might,
the reluctance to rebel, put up a fight.
But women, by and large, have no choice,
for those like me, who raise their voice,
to question mothers-in-law and misters,
fare far worse than their submissive sisters.
But the last ounce of strength I'll gather,
and whip the horses of my will to lather.
If I can light a flame in but one woman,
I'll consider my work on this earth done,
for when I falter and fall, others will rise
to carry my torch towards a new sunrise.

2

Sex across Cultures

Perspectives on sex differ significantly among various cultures. They range from severe repression to permissiveness bordering on promiscuity. Eastern countries such as China, Iran, and India value chastity in a potential mate, making premarital sex a definite 'no'. The hymen is considered sacrosanct, to be broken only by a woman's lawfully wedded husband. It is seen as a symbol of her moral standing and, tragically, of her worth if she is unfortunate enough to end up in the flesh trade.

Unmarried girls who have had sexual relations often resort to bizarre methods to pretend to be virgins. Some insert a cotton swab soaked in the blood of a freshly beheaded fowl, usually procured by their lover, into their vagina. Those who have access to, and can afford, medical intervention undergo hymenoplasty (revirgination), a minor surgical procedure, before being wed to a stranger of their parents' choice.

An unusual film, *Leeches*, tells the story of a sister who saves her younger sibling from becoming a one-day bride to a middle-aged Sheikh—sex with a virgin is believed to cure syphilis—by taking her place. Though the elder sister has a lover, she applies leeches to her vagina so that she can pretend to be a virgin. This sordid practice is reportedly still prevalent in poorer quarters of Hyderabad, where a father of many daughters sacrifices one to a wealthy Sheikh from the Gulf so that he can use the money obtained to settle the others.[2]

Conversely, cultures with less gender discrimination, such as those in the West, are more tolerant of sex before marriage, with the Netherlands being among the most permissive. Sex education begins in early primary school and is a compulsory part of the school curriculum. Media restrictions on sexual imagery are minimal. Contrary to popular expectation, this permissive attitude has helped the country avoid many major issues associated with sexuality. Sweden has among the lowest rates of teenage pregnancy and sexually transmitted diseases in the world.[3]

Despite these benefits, even countries such as the United States are not uniformly progressive in their views on sex. France is relatively more open, while Ireland is less so. Russians and Filipinos tend to look down upon sex before the age of sixteen. Attitudes can also vary widely within a single country. However, women across the world continue to resort to prostitution for economic reasons, as their sexuality is often all they have to sell.

The extremes of sexual attitudes were studied by anthropologists working in isolated regions of the world. In 1966, anthropologist John Cowan Messenger found that Inis Beag, a small island off the coast of Ireland, had extremely restrictive sexual behaviour. Nudity was not tolerated—adults washed only those parts of their bodies visible outside their clothes—and married couples kept their undergarments on during sex. The husband initiated the act, with minimal foreplay, performed it in the missionary position, reached orgasm quickly, and fell asleep. Female orgasm was almost unheard of. Sex was believed to be physically taxing for men, and couples refrained from intercourse on the night before a hard day's work.

In sharp contrast, anthropologist Donald S. Marshall found the people of Mangaia Island in the South Pacific to be extremely promiscuous. Sexual knowledge began at the age of seven, while both boys and girls had sexual encounters by the age of thirteen. At this age, a boy underwent an incision along the entire length of the upper part of the penis. The expert who performed the procedure also provided detailed instructions about sex. Two weeks after this rite of passage, the boy had intercourse with an experienced woman who taught him various acts and positions and, more importantly, how to delay orgasm so that both partners experienced pleasure at the same time. Young girls received similar instruction, and both sexes were encouraged to have numerous sexual encounters with different partners before marriage. Men learnt that bringing a woman to orgasm was one of their prime sources of pleasure. As a result, unlike the people of Inis Beag, the people of Mangaia reportedly did not suffer from stress and anxiety.

Somewhere between these extremes lies Mehinaku, a village in central Brazil that appears to have abundant sex as well as anxiety. Sex is free and open, but myths warn that people who have sex outside marriage die in fantastic ways. There is little understanding of orgasm, menstruation is believed to be dangerous, and gender segregation is strictly enforced. A woman who breaks this rule risks being gang-raped in the woods. Despite these contradictions and fears, sexual relationships are actively sought and indulged in.

These studies were conducted decades ago, and there is no way of knowing whether people in these remote areas have since been exposed to mainstream culture and changed accordingly.

Turning to what is considered normal sexual behaviour in the modern world, region and religion continue to play a significant role. Islam, Buddhism, Hinduism, and Catholicism encourage chastity and abstinence while looking down upon promiscuity. Masculine cultures such as ours uphold double standards: Men are allowed to sow wild oats, while women are expected to remain 'pure'.

In yogic philosophy, Brahmacharya—that includes control over thoughts, speech, and physical celibacy—is believed to cultivate mental and spiritual growth by transmuting sexual energy into *Ojas* (spiritual energy). This, in turn, reduces stress, enhances intelligence, focus, willpower, calm, concentration, and cognition

Acculturation also plays a significant role in ethnic differences. Acculturation refers to the process by which individuals from minority ethnic groups incorporate two layers of culture—that of their heritage and that of the mainstream—into their self-identity. This usually occurs over generations, as an ethnic group gradually loses some characteristics of its heritage culture while adopting those of the dominant culture.

First-generation immigrants from India living in the West may acquire girlfriends or boyfriends and engage in live-in relationships, which they hide from conservative parents back home. When the time for marriage arrives, many return to India to meekly marry spouses chosen by their parents: Boys seek virgins with fat dowries, while girls opt for the perceived stability of arranged marriages after experiencing the insecurities of foreign love affairs. Recent immigrants tend to be more conservative than second-generation non-resident Indians, whose attitudes towards sex often change along with their sartorial choices. Over time, they begin to behave like the community they are now part of.

An interesting study conducted by Tierney K. Arnold and Cindy M. Meston between 2001 and 2004 examined 'Ethnic Differences in Sexual Attitudes of U.S. College Students: Gender, Acculturation, and Religiosity Factors'. The researchers studied sexual attitudes among Euro-American, Asian, and Hispanic American college students, focusing on the merging of heritage and mainstream cultures and the role of religion. A total of 1,415 students (67 per cent Euro-American, 16 per cent Hispanic, and 17 per cent Asian; 32 per cent men and 68 per cent women) completed a questionnaire covering four key areas of sexual attitudes:

- Attitudes towards homosexuality, which predict gender equality, sexual knowledge, and comfort
- Attitudes towards casual sex, where liberal views predict a higher risk of sexually transmitted diseases
- Attitudes towards gender-role traditionality, which predict marriage practices, the importance of sexual pleasure for women, and attitudes towards pregnancy and contraception
- Attitudes towards extramarital sex, reflecting the acceptability of sexuality outside marriage

As expected, Asian participants were more conservative than Hispanic participants, who leaned closer to Euro-American sexual behaviour. However, higher levels of acculturation—particularly among those born in the United States—were associated with sexual attitudes more similar to Euro-American counterparts. Those with strong religious or spiritual beliefs were less likely to abandon traditional views. Ethnic groups abroad also tend to live together and perpetuate their own culture, building places of worship and celebrating religious festivals and marriages, often following rituals more ardently than their counterparts in India. Meanwhile, their children are exposed to liberal attitudes towards sexuality at school and college. This dichotomy creates stress, as they long to merge rather than stand out. To satisfy both parents and peers, many engage in sexual activity while hiding it from conservative families.

Between total acculturation and rigid adherence to one's heritage culture lies a large bicultural diaspora. Here, individuals integrate elements of the mainstream culture while maintaining strong ties to their roots. At the far end are religious fundamentalists, who believe in absolute religious authority and reject ideological intermingling—sexual or otherwise. In summary, the young are more inclined to assimilate, the older generation tends to be bicultural, and fanatics remain resistant to change.

3

What Women Really Want in Bed

Human sexuality is the way people express themselves sexually. It encompasses our sexual feelings, thoughts, and behaviours—an amalgam of biological, erotic, physical, and emotional conditioning. Though procreation is the goal of sexual intercourse in the animal world (and humans are no exception), people also have sex with those to whom they are physically attracted, as a means to a very pleasurable end. It also deepens emotional connection.

Sexual stirrings begin at puberty and continue throughout life, even after menopause. Children, too, find pleasure in touching their genitalia. While masculine sexual desire and its satisfaction are overt and socially acceptable, female sexuality has been kept under wraps for centuries. It is time the world realises that women are sexual beings, too. Instead of suppressing their sexuality, as has long been done because of socio-religious conditioning, girls should be told that sex is beautiful—provided it is experienced with the right partner at the right time. The expression of female sexuality should be empowering, not demeaning, but the reality is often quite different.

Instead of celebrating our sexuality and acknowledging that we are equal partners in intimate relationships, we allow ourselves to be regarded as objects of masculine sexual desire. So deeply are we conditioned to objectify ourselves that, often subconsciously, we dress and behave in ways meant to arouse a man's desire, when we should be voicing our own. From their teens, girls are subjected to the indignity of eve-teasing. Though horrified by catcalls and unwanted touching, a tiny part of our minds may enjoy the attention because it reiterates our desirability to members of the opposite sex. At times, revelling in the power it gives us over men, we may even use our sexuality to our advantage.

We have been led to believe that only 'bad girls' like sex. How, then, do we change this mindset? The first step towards a sexually fulfilling life—and there is nothing more fulfilling—is to believe that sex and orgasm are the birthright of every woman. Sexual health is as important as physical, mental, and emotional health to overall well-being, so do not let false notions of modesty stand in the way. However, it is important to remember that sex is not only about pleasure. The dangers of unsafe sex are many and can have lifelong repercussions on sexual and reproductive health. Consent is of paramount importance; moreover, sex with a girl under eighteen years of age is considered rape under the law, even if she gives her consent.

Once we accept that we are sexual beings, too, we must have candid conversations with our partners about our needs and satisfaction. This is easier said than done, as most of us are too embarrassed or inhibited to speak openly. Many men are horrified or disgusted by the audacity of a woman making such requests or demands. Only an occasional, considerate partner understands and obliges. Once these hurdles are crossed, heaven is within reach. All one has to do is seize it.

Another preconceived notion is that love automatically leads to good sex. This is not always true. While it certainly helps to be in love with one's partner, a couple must still work towards discovering each other's erogenous zones—areas that, when stimulated, lead to arousal and orgasm.

Let me tell you the story of a couple madly in love, yet a terrible disappointment to each other in bed.

Malini married her childhood sweetheart, Mohit. To finally be with him night and day ought to have been sheer bliss, but it was not. She had yet to experience the sexual ecstasy so often spoken of and was deeply disappointed. Like any 'good girl', she was a virgin before marriage, but now, contrary to her expectations, she found no pleasure in the act. Though Mohit ejaculated night after night, he derived little joy from the union, for he gave no joy to his beloved wife. She felt bad for making him feel bad and dreaded their futile nightly endeavours.

Matters escalated to such an extent that the lovey-dovey couple, once considered adorable by the entire college during their courtship, were barely on speaking terms. It affected Mohit's work, and his colleagues began to notice. One day, his best friend, Ronit, confronted him.

'Where has the fun-loving, happy-go-lucky Mohit gone? I miss him, yaar.'

After some persuasion, Mohit broke down and confessed his nightly fiascos.

'Why don't you ask her what she wants you to do?' Ronit suggested.

'Is it that simple?'

'It is. If you can't talk to each other about something as important as this, what's the use of being married?'

'But what if she doesn't cooperate?'

'No harm in trying. If it doesn't work, you can always seek professional help.'

Mohit drove home in a pensive mood. He decided not to have sex with Malini until she indicated, by word or sign, that she wanted it. Determined to bring some joy back into their lives, he shook off his melancholy at the door and surprised her with a cheerful smile.

'Let's go out on a date and relive our days of courtship,' he whispered.

This sent a tingle down her spine; after all, foreplay begins long before a couple gets into bed.

'If only we could,' Malini muttered under her breath, but because she loved him, she agreed.

Soon they were seated at their favourite table in their favourite restaurant, served by their favourite waiter. Despite herself, Malini regained her good humour, especially when Mohit tucked a string of jasmine into her hair. On the way back home, however, the good feeling began to ebb, for she dreaded the currency with which she would have to pay for the lovely evening.

I'll try my best not to tense up while he is at it. Perhaps I could fake an orgasm, she thought, though she had no idea how to.

Back home, to her surprise, the romance continued without the abrasive intrusion of sex. Mohit had the good sense not to force her. He lay beside her, held her hand, and spoke of old times, reiterating his love. It was the closest Malini had come to bliss. She gave him a fleeting kiss of gratitude and turned the other way so they could sleep spooned together, her favourite position.

Half asleep, Mohit flung his arm across her chest, his fingertips lightly brushing her breast through her flimsy nightgown. Her nipples hardened, giving rise to stirrings hitherto unknown. She wanted him to take her but felt too embarrassed to ask.

The next night, to his surprise, she seemed more receptive, but he dared not hurry and risk another disaster. They lay side by side, his arm under her neck, his hand playing with her ear. She found this strangely erotic and would have responded had he continued, but to her surprise, he went no further.

'Is something wrong?' she asked.

'Why do you ask?'

'It's just that you . . . you . . .' She could not muster the courage to finish the sentence.

'I don't seem to please you in bed, no matter how hard I try.'

She tensed, which made him tense. He withdrew his arm and rolled over, frustrated by the futility of his efforts. This sudden withdrawal made Malini contrite. He was trying, and she was not helping him at all.

'It's not that I don't . . .' Her voice trailed off.

'If there is anything you want me to do, you only have to tell me.'

True. How was he to know if she would not speak? All she could manage was, 'I can't.'

'Why?'

'I feel shy.'

He was incredulous; they had known each other all their lives. 'Then how will I know?'

Just as he began to despair, an idea struck him. 'Let's play a game.'

'A game?'

'I'll blindfold you and run my fingers over your body. Just nod when it feels good. If you're too shy even for that, I'll know by your expressions what turns you on and what doesn't.'

She nodded, blushing happily. And thus, it happened that Malini experienced her first climax that night—and a mind-blowing one at that. After that, there was no stopping the lovebirds, who turned into enthusiastic explorers of the land of ecstasy. Though Malini and Mohit's story had a happy conclusion, or rather, a new beginning that lasted a lifetime, many couples are not so fortunate.

What Women Want in Bed

Questionnaires answered anonymously by thousands of women revealed what they genuinely wanted. While personal preferences varied, by and large, women reported a better sexual experience with partners with whom they felt an emotional connection. They liked to be wooed and made to feel special—romance never goes out of style. Almost all preferred a slow build-up, though an occasional 'quickie' could be gratifying. Some women enjoyed pressure or stimulation of the mons pubis, though the majority required clitoral stimulation to climax. Staying power was appreciated but not essential. A partner who brought her to the brink before penetration did not need prolonged intercourse to satisfy her, as she was already primed for orgasm. Some liked dirty talk; others did not. Some enjoyed a noisy partner or vocalised themselves, while others found this off-putting.

Sexual Blueprints

Sexual compatibility does not mean liking the same things. It means each partner understands what makes the other feel good and invests time and effort in mutual pleasure. Sex therapists have found that everybody—male or female—has a distinct sexual blueprint.

An *energetic* type responds to anticipation: A hovering hand, a near-touch, the light brushing of body hair. A *sensual* type requires stimulation of the senses—smell, sight, sound, touch, taste—individually or together. A *sexual* type is aroused by thoughts of nudity, genitals, penetration, and intercourse. A *kinky* type is aroused by what is taboo. Finally, the *shapeshifter* may be turned on by any or all of the above.

Couples may also indulge in body mapping, during which one partner explores the other's body—blindfolded or not—rating each touch on a scale of one to five. The partner being touched actively surrenders and offers feedback rather than lying passively. The combinations are endless, and each couple must discover what works best for them. Knowing what arouses one's partner is, in itself, deeply arousing.

Innovation

One important truth to remember is this: Couples who innovate last. No matter how sexually enthusiastic a couple is at the beginning, ennui eventually creeps in. Sex with the same partner can become routine, predictable, and dull. This must be addressed to prevent emotional distance or infidelity.

Couples should consciously make an effort to revitalise their sex lives. They might pretend to meet as strangers at a bar, flirt, talk smut, and book a hotel room for a one-night stand. One partner could play the innocent, the other the initiator. They might indulge in role play—cop and criminal, teacher and student, boss and secretary. A candlelit massage, sex in different settings, or consensual experimentation can go a long way in keeping intimacy alive. All it takes is time, willingness, and desire.

Communication remains the single most crucial factor in resolving dissatisfaction or cold wars in bed. How can your partner know what you want if you do not tell him? Contrary to popular belief, he cannot read your mind. You must voice your likes and dislikes, desires and aversions, however embarrassing it may feel. If he is caring and considerate, he will respond to your mutual satisfaction.

Alternatively, couples can read a book on sexuality or watch an erotic film together and use it as a starting point for conversation, gradually introducing personal preferences. Avoid pressurising each other to achieve orgasm; it is counterproductive. Enjoy touching, kissing, and cuddling, for sex is not only physical but deeply emotional. If, despite genuine effort, a couple remains unable to resolve their sexual difficulties, it is time to seek professional help.

4

The Female Orgasm

When asked, 'Where are a person's sex organs situated?' people tend to state the obvious: 'Between the legs.' The correct answer, however, is 'between the ears,' for the brain is the biggest sex organ. Only when desire arises in the brain—whatever the stimulus, be it visual, olfactory, imagery, or memory—does it send signals to the genitalia to prepare for the act through lubrication, engorgement, and erection, and, if the time and place are right, take it to its logical conclusion, either with a partner or through self-stimulation.

Orgasm

'An orgasm is a physical reflex that occurs when muscles tighten during sexual arousal and then relax through a series of rhythmic contractions.' It is the most pleasurable sensation a human being can experience. While much has been said about the male orgasm, the female orgasm remains something of a mystery. Male orgasm leads to the release of semen and serves a clear biological function—reproduction—while the function of the female orgasm is less clearly defined. It is not necessary for impregnation, as rape victims can conceive. Perhaps the intense pleasure experienced during orgasm encourages a woman to engage in sex and thereby contributes indirectly to procreation.

More often than not, sex is indulged in as a recreational activity. Satisfactory sex and orgasm promote bonding, reduce stress, boost immunity, induce a sense of well-being, and improve sleep.

They lower blood pressure, improve heart health and self-esteem, decrease anxiety, stress, and depression, and provide immediate natural pain relief. Orgasm also increases pain threshold, which may explain why spanking or hair pulling can result in what some describe as 'good pain'. Some doctors even advocate climaxing during childbirth to decrease the intensity of labour pains, though one is hardly inclined towards such activity at that time. Orgasmic sexual activity after waking up can be energising, making sex a pleasurable form of exercise.

Studies have shown that women who have sex at least once a week tend to have more regular menstrual cycles, though this may or may not boost fertility. There is little scientific evidence to prove that orgasm improves skin, hair, or overall health, though there is often a visible glow on the face of a woman who has just climaxed.

Stages of Sexual Response

The female sexual response begins with the excitement phase, which may last from several minutes to several hours. During this phase, heart rate, blood pressure, and respiration increase. The skin becomes flushed due to increased blood supply to the surface. Distensible parts of the body, such as the nipples and clitoris, swell. Increased blood flow to the genitals leads to engorgement and heightened sensitivity, the vagina expands, and genital fluids are secreted.

This is followed by a brief plateau phase, during which maximal arousal is maintained. Orgasm is marked by sudden, intense pleasure and rhythmic muscle spasms in the vagina, often accompanied by involuntary sounds. It lasts only a few seconds, after which the woman enters the resolution phase—a state of deep relaxation and return to normal or even subnormal physiological levels.

Up to this point, the sexual response sequence in men and women is similar. After orgasm, however, the male enters a refractory phase, during which he is unresponsive to sexual stimulation. The female, in contrast, may continue to respond to stimulation and experience multiple orgasms without entering a refractory phase.

Women are more likely to orgasm if they are in a loving relationship, especially if their partner expresses love during sex, if they are asked what they want in bed, if sexual activity is prolonged, if they try new positions or locations, or if their sexual fantasies are enacted. Prolonged foreplay increases desire and pleasure and may begin long before bedtime through suggestive messages, a phone call from a partner at work, knowing glances, double-meaning words or sentences, subtle gestures, or a surreptitious touch under the dinner table in a room full of people. All of this builds sexual tension, leading to intense arousal and gratifying sex when the couple finally comes together.

It is not always possible to tell whether a woman has had an orgasm. Some moan or make guttural sounds, others cling to their partner until the contractions subside, while some flush or perspire. If unsure, a partner need only ask gently whether she is satisfied. If not, it does not necessarily mean his efforts were inadequate. He may help her achieve satisfaction through manual stimulation of her genitals.

Good and Bad Orgasms

This brings us to the distinction between a good orgasm and a bad one. A bad orgasm may result purely from physical stimulation, without desire or emotional connection. A woman may feel obligated to climax to please her partner or simply to get it over with. Fatigue, stress, illness, medication, and sleep deprivation are major contributory factors. Other factors include an abusive partner or one to whom she is not physically attracted, as often happens in arranged marriages. While orgasm may still occur, it brings no joy. Even forced sex can trigger orgasm when specific points are stimulated, but it is never pleasurable.

Orgasm may occur during heterosexual or homosexual contact (it is said to be more intense among lesbians), masturbation, mutual masturbation, the use of sex toys, or during wet dreams. One may climax while exercising or while watching others have sex, whether in real life or pornography. Orgasms may also be induced by stimulation of the nipples, clitoris, vagina, anus, or all of these together—a blended orgasm.

Clitoral Orgasm

Clitoral orgasm is the most common form of female orgasm, as the clitoris is an extremely sensitive part of a woman's anatomy, containing thousands of nerve endings. Touching, caressing, or stroking it—directly or indirectly, in up-and-down or circular motions—increases blood flow to the area, leading to engorgement and release. Some women prefer a light touch; others enjoy firm pressure. It takes time and attentiveness to understand an individual woman's clitoris.

Artist Sophia Wallace held an exhibition at the Leslie-Lohman Museum in New York titled *Cliteracy* to enlighten the world about this little jewel hidden deep within a woman—one capable of giving more pleasure than all the diamonds in the world.

The word 'clitoris' comes from the Greek *kleitoris*, meaning 'key'; it is indeed the key to feminine ecstasy. Wallace famously stated that 'the clitoris is not a button, it's an iceberg,' as only a small portion is externally visible. Its actual length is approximately four inches, three-quarters of which lies beneath the surface. Only the head and hood are visible; the shaft is internal. Some believe the G-spot is part of the clitoral structure.

The clitoris varies in size and shape among women. Some are hidden beneath the hood; others protrude. It grows throughout a woman's life and may become up to two and a half times larger after menopause, leading to stronger orgasms in some women. Women who have given birth often have a larger clitoris. It contains about 8,000 nerve endings; roughly double those found in the glans of the penis. As a result, an average clitoral orgasm often lasts longer than the most intense male orgasm, involving anywhere from three to sixteen contractions lasting ten to thirty seconds.

A 2023-study reported 10,281 nerve fibres in the clitoris, making it the most nerve-rich part of the human body.[4]

Vaginal Orgasm

A vaginal orgasm occurs after vaginal penetration, with or without clitoral stimulation. Not all women experience vaginal orgasms, and there is nothing abnormal about this, contrary to Freud's claim that vaginal orgasm is superior or more mature. No evidence supports this view.

The G-spot, or Gräfenberg spot, has been studied since the 1940s, though disagreement persists regarding its existence and precise location. It is said to be an extension of the clitoris, located on the anterior vaginal wall, two to three inches from the vaginal opening. Some researchers suggest it is not a distinct spot but an area. When stimulated, it may lead to intense orgasms and, in some cases, female ejaculation.

Women who experience vaginal orgasms are more likely to have thicker tissue in the anterior vaginal wall. Those attempting to locate the G-spot may insert a forefinger into the vagina, curl it forward, and gently explore the anterior wall until a sensitive area is found, often at the junction of the ridged and smooth tissue. Direct stimulation of this area may result in orgasms more intense than those achieved through clitoral stimulation alone. It is not easily accessible during intercourse without specific angles or positions. Special sex toys, such as curved G-spot vibrators, may enhance stimulation.

Misled by pornography and other unreliable sources, some women seek a dubious procedure called G-spot amplification. After numbing the area with local anaesthesia, collagen or other substances are injected beneath the vaginal skin. This procedure has been disapproved by the American College of Obstetricians and Gynaecologists as neither safe nor effective. It may cause scarring, adhesions, and painful intercourse, defeating its very purpose.

If locating the G-spot were not challenging enough, other erogenous areas have been described: The A-spot on the upper anterior vaginal wall beneath the cervix; the O-spot on the posterior wall behind the cervix. Stimulation of the upper vagina may cause pleasurable uterine contractions, leading to what is known as a cervical orgasm.

PS-spot is located in the perineal body, the area between the vagina and anus. It has a rich nerve and blood supply, as it anchors the various muscles of the pelvic floor. An intact perineal body is crucial for maintaining adequate tone for proper sexual sensation and satisfaction. Damage after childbirth—tears or episiotomies—impacts postpartum sexual health, resulting in decreased libido and sexual satisfaction. It requires rehabilitation of the pelvic floor, muscle training, and massage.

There is, however, no need to turn sex—a deeply pleasurable activity—into a clinical exercise, nor to feel disappointed if climax is achieved only through clitoral stimulation. For those unable to locate spots whose existence remains scientifically uncertain, it is best to let go of the elusive. There is no need to feel sexually inadequate. Enjoy what feels good rather than yearning for what may not exist. Thousands of women have never experienced orgasm, and many men struggle with premature ejaculation; compared to this, one has much to be grateful for.

Blended Orgasm

A blended orgasm occurs when more than one erogenous zone—usually the clitoris and vagina—is stimulated simultaneously. This may be achieved through masturbation, sex toys, or with a partner stimulating the G-spot while also stimulating the clitoris manually or orally. Positions such as cowgirl, reverse cowgirl, standing, spooning, closed missionary, or modified doggy style allow access to both areas. Blended orgasms may also involve nipple or anal stimulation alongside vaginal penetration.

Anal Orgasm

Sexual activity should always centre on what brings pleasure and comfort. Not all women enjoy anal sex, and no one should ever be coerced into it. However, for those curious to explore, it is useful to know that the anus and rectum share nerves and muscles with the vagina and clitoris. Anal stimulation, whether with fingers or penile penetration, may result in orgasm.

Butt plugs are sex toys designed for insertion into the rectum. They must be well-lubricated and inserted gently. They resemble dildos but are shorter and have a flanged base to prevent them from being drawn into the rectum, which connects to the digestive tract and may require surgical removal if an object is lost. No such risk exists with vaginal insertion of sex toys, as the cervix blocks the upper end of the vagina. Butt plugs should be covered with a condom for hygiene and protection against infections. Even when covered, they should never be shared.

Nipple Orgasm

Nipples are a major erogenous zone and play a key role in sexual arousal. When touched, stroked, kissed, or sucked, they become erect due to their rich nerve supply and sensitive skin. Some women are able to climax through breast fondling and nipple stimulation alone.

Exercise Orgasm

Some women experience orgasms during physical workouts, often referred to as 'coregasms', as they commonly occur during core-strengthening exercises. Kegel exercises, which involve tightening and relaxing the pelvic floor muscles, may evoke sexual sensations that result in orgasm, with or without direct clitoral or vaginal stimulation.

Sleep Orgasm

Some women experience orgasm during an erotic (wet) dream, just as men have 'night-falls' (involuntary ejaculation during sleep). This is entirely normal, and there is no need to feel embarrassed about it. While on the subject, a brief mention of 'sexsomnia' would not be out of place.

Sexsomnia is a sleep disorder in which a person may masturbate or attempt to have sex with the individual lying next to them while asleep. The person is unaware of their actions and has no recollection of them upon waking. Being caught masturbating in one's sleep or grabbing the person beside you can be deeply embarrassing or traumatic for the other person.

These episodes can be reduced by improving sleep quality, lowering stress levels, reducing night-time alcohol or drug consumption, and having more conscious sexual activity—in short, by eliminating known triggers. The person sleeping next to her may gently push her away or simply not respond. If such episodes are infrequent, treatment is usually unnecessary; otherwise, consultation with a sleep specialist is advised. Certain psychiatric medications may help by increasing deep sleep.

While discussing psychological issues related to sex, it is worth mentioning post-sex sadness, a condition some women experience. Medically termed post-coital dysphoria (PCD), it is characterised by intense feelings of sadness, anger, or distress after sex—often following satisfying sex and orgasm—which may reduce a woman to tears. No definitive cause has been identified, though hormonal fluctuations, prior sexual trauma, or guilt following extramarital sex may play a role. If post-sex blues become overwhelming or interfere with one's sex life, therapy is recommended. Some women may also experience post-sex headaches or migraines, which may or may not require treatment depending on severity.

Multiple Orgasms: A Female Advantage

Women are biologically endowed with the ability to experience multiple orgasms in succession, whereas men require a refractory period between ejaculations before another erection and climax are possible. This is because women do not experience a refractory period after orgasm. Not all women may achieve multiple orgasms, but those who wish to may find it helpful to keep their pelvic muscles contracted to maintain the plateau phase, making it easier to reach subsequent climaxes.

Edging: The Art of Delay

Edging is a sexual practice that deliberately delays orgasm. This is achieved by reducing thrusting or 'cooling down' just before climax, allowing the urge to subside before starting again. The process is repeated until the desire for orgasm becomes almost unbearable, culminating in an explosive release. This technique has long been practised by Tantric adepts in India, who are said to sustain sexual activity for as long as two hours.

Do Women Ejaculate?

Meena and I were gynaecologists at the same hospital and close friends. Beyond professional discussions, our late-evening walks often led to intimate conversations. My recently published book, *For the Love of a Man*, candidly revealed details of an extramarital affair pursued in search of an orgasm that had eluded me within my marriage—an affair that resulted in multiple orgasms and sordid repercussions. Though the rift in my marriage could never be fully repaired, and though my lover ultimately proved unworthy of my affections, I have no regrets, whatever the price I paid. I shudder to think that I might have lived and died without experiencing the ecstasy my body was capable of. I shudder even more at the desperation with which I once sought a divorce—to marry a man whose sole redeeming quality was his sexuality.

After the book's release, a strange phenomenon occurred. Female acquaintances began confiding secrets of their sex lives they would never have shared otherwise. They knew I would not judge them, as I was hardly in a position to do so. The knowledge gained planted the seed for this book on female sexuality. Meena was one such confidante.

She was a tall, angular woman in her early forties. Though she had two children, she blossomed sexually rather late—much like me—but with her husband. With their children away at boarding school, they had the house to themselves. One evening, while watching a blue film together, her arousal was so intense that it culminated in a mind-blowing orgasm. A copious amount of fluid gushed from her genitals, soaking the bedsheet.

'It must be urine,' I said.

'I swear it wasn't. I had emptied my bladder beforehand and felt no urge.'

'Then what could it be?' I asked, puzzled.

I was familiar with excessive lubrication during foreplay—some highly orgasmic women literally drip in anticipation, much to their partner's discomfort, but this was something else.

Determined to repeat the experience, Meena ensured that every weekend her husband rested in the afternoon so he would be fresh for the prolonged session at night; it took her nearly two hours to reach that state of bliss. Eventually, they took to placing a thickly folded bedsheet beneath her to contain the exquisite gush of fluid.

I could make neither head nor tail of it. Sadly, such phenomena are not taught in medical college, and I had never encountered it before. I believed myself an expert after years with my accomplished lover, yet this had never occurred between us.

It was only while researching for this book that I came across the term 'female ejaculation'. Simply put, it refers to the expulsion of fluid through the urethra during or before orgasm. Colloquially known as squirting or gushing, it may range from a few drops to a forceful stream soaking the bedsheets.

As early as the sixteenth century, it was noted that the female 'draws forth the man's seed and casts her own with it.'[5] In the seventeenth century, experts wrote of the female urethra releasing 'great quantities of saline liquor during coition, which increases the heat and enjoyment of women.' In 1918, anarchist Almeda Sperry described to her lesbian partner the 'rhythmic spurt of your love juices.'

In Rwanda-Rundi and parts of Uganda and Tanzania, there exists a practice called *Kunyaza*. The word means 'to urinate', though it also refers to female ejaculation. Its origins are said to be serendipitous. In the third century, a queen reportedly took a guard as her lover. Overcome by performance anxiety, he stimulated her vulva and clitoris rather than penetrating her—an act that resulted in intense pleasure. *Kunyaza* is now practised to enhance mutual pleasure and induce female ejaculation.

In this practice, the male partner first taps and rubs the outer surface of the labia minora with his organ, then its inner surface. After this, he proceeds to stimulate the vulval vestibule—the space enclosed between the two labia minora (which includes the clitoris and urinary and vaginal openings) in a similar manner. As the woman's pubic hair might come in the way, it is removed beforehand. After she has been sufficiently aroused, he penetrates her, alternating shallow thrusts barely past her vaginal opening and deep thrusts right up to the cervix, all the while making circular movements with his organ that he holds between his middle and index fingers. This results in an intense orgasm and female ejaculation, sometimes even before her partner.

Researchers believe that female ejaculation and squirting are two distinct processes that may occur together during orgasm. Squirting involves the sudden expulsion of liquid, from the bladder and containing urine, whereas ejaculate is a milky-white fluid secreted by the Skene's (paraurethral) glands into the urethra. It is called *saspanda nadi* in the Indian sex manual *Ananga Ranga*, a manual that predates the *Kama Sutra*. Skene's glands are the female equivalent of the prostate, located in the anterior vaginal wall near the G-spot. During arousal, they swell and release fluid that aids lubrication and protects against urinary tract infections (UTIs); at times, this fluid may be copious enough to resemble ejaculation.

It is important to note that most women with normal sexual function do not ejaculate. Watching women squirt in pornography can make others feel inadequate, which is neither accurate nor desirable. There is no evidence linking female ejaculation to better sex, so one should neither chase nor fear it . . . simply enjoy the experience.

On one side are women who desire such an experience; on the other are those who ejaculate but feel ashamed of it. The sensation of needing to urinate before ejaculation causes some women to suppress climax for fear of 'wetting' their partner. Others avoid sexual intimacy altogether, mistakenly believing that such an occurrence is abhorrent and seek medical help for what is, in fact, a natural variation.

Pelvic Massage: A Curious History

I would like to conclude this discussion by touching upon pelvic massage, a practice prevalent in Europe and America during the nineteenth and early twentieth centuries.

Sexually dissatisfied women in the Victorian era were diagnosed with 'hysteria', for which a physician would be summoned. Treatment involved pelvic massage, including clitoral stimulation, culminating in what was termed a 'hysterical paroxysm'—an orgasm believed to relieve symptoms such as headaches, fatigue, and depression.

Manual pelvic massage proved taxing for physicians, leading to the invention of clitoral vibrators. As the saying goes, necessity is the mother of invention. While one might assume such work to have been titillating, perhaps the physical strain and the emotional toll of providing release without receiving it proved otherwise. However, physicians did lament the advent of the stethoscope; before its invention, they pressed their ears directly to women's bosoms to listen to heart and lung sounds.

Today, pelvic massage has re-emerged as a clinical practice, administered by trained professionals. This is not equivalent to 'pelvic massage' for sexual stimulation; rather, it is a conservative therapeutic strategy to manage pelvic floor dysfunction.

5

Self-Gratification

A young housekeeping staff member was cleaning up the room in a five-star hotel after a distinguished guest vacated it. As was the protocol, she opened the locker to look for valuables inadvertently left behind. Imagine her surprise when she saw an obscene-looking pink object in it. Before the bewildered girl could decide what to make of it, it started vibrating! She gave a little scream and stepped back.

The duty manager was duly called. He realised that it was a dildo, something the poor girl had never seen in her life! It so happened that the lady who left it behind was a valued customer, the CEO of a company that gave them good business. She must have been disturbed in the midst of a pleasurable session with the 'object of her desire' and had to quickly put it in the locker without switching it off, hence the intermittent gasps of a dying battery!

Hotels have to be discreet in handling such delicate matters. Off went an e-mail informing the lady of the 'pink object' found in her locker, asking her if they should courier it to her address. She was in her forties and had married late. Horrified at the thought of her husband receiving the parcel, she sent an immediate reply: 'Dispose, dispose, dispose.'

To which they replied, 'Disposed, disposed, disposed.'

The matter was satisfactorily settled. Whenever their paths crossed, the duty manager would plague the poor housekeeping girl with the playful query, 'Have you found any more pink objects?'

Most people would be unsympathetic towards the CEO who managed the company with a no-nonsense air in the boardroom and indulged in such obscene activities in her bedroom; however, such a judgement would be unkind.

No matter what men would like to believe, women, too, are sexual beings; what is she to do when the urge arises? Invite a stranger to her room, and with him invite a load of trouble that could take the form of blackmail or STIs? Masturbation, by whatever means, is the safest way of relieving sexual tension.

When my husband passed away, a US-based cousin, coming to India on a visit, offered to bring me solace in the form of a vibrator!

'Please don't!' I exclaimed. 'I wouldn't be caught dead with it. Alive, perhaps I might have considered . . .'

'What do you mean?'

'I dread the thought of my children finding it by my bed after my death.'

Sadly, even adult children rarely come to terms with their parents' sexuality.

⚤

A young girl came to me with a history of itching in the genital area and discharge. I asked her if she was sexually active.

'Yes,' she replied.

'Get your partner treated, too, as you can get reinfected.'

'I don't have a boyfriend.'

'But you just said . . .' I asked, perplexed.

'I pleasure myself.'

'Oh! Do you insert anything inside?' I asked, after I recovered my composure.

'Only my fingers.'

'Then cut your nails,' I said, prescribing the requisite medication.

Masturbation is the sexual stimulation of one's own genitals for sexual pleasure that usually ends in orgasm. It is derived from the Latin verb *masturbari*, which is a corrupted form of the words *manu stuprare*, meaning 'to defile with the hand'. There are depictions of male and female masturbation in prehistoric rock paintings; animals masturbate, so do divine creatures, if mythology is to be believed.

Most of us have masturbated at some time or another. It is frequent in both sexes and at any age, right from early childhood. Babies in cribs enjoy playing with their genitals, as do toddlers and small children.[6] An Italian doctor even demonstrated a female foetus masturbating *in utero*! This pleasurable activity continues through adolescence and adulthood, right up to middle age and beyond. Some people masturbate often (several times a day, a week, or a month), while others rarely, and yet others don't masturbate at all. How often a person masturbates is not a problem unless it interferes with day-to-day life.

Different people masturbate in different ways. It is usually done by rubbing with the hand, the use of fingers, or hand showers for clitoral stimulation. Fingers, firm elongated objects, or sex toys are inserted in the vagina. There is no 'normal' way of masturbation.

Fantasy plays an important part, and women often imagine themselves having sex with some celebrity (Brad Pitt is a hot favourite) or with a person she is keen on. Masturbation also relieves the sexual tension generated by reading or watching pornography.

Myths Associated with Masturbation

Though the pleasure is intense, it is usually followed by a feeling of shame or guilt, especially in misinformed young adults. This could lead to psychological problems, for there are horrific myths associated with masturbation. The gullible fall prey to these misconceptions and endure immense torture. Unable to control the urge, they indulge again and, fearing the repercussions, flagellate themselves with the whip of self-reproach, and the vicious cycle continues.

Myths are often propagated by quacks posing as 'sex specialists' because people seeking a cure for self-gratification form a major part of their practice. They have the gullible believe that masturbation could cause weakness, insanity, blindness, impotence, penis shrinkage or curvature, unsatisfactory sexual relationships, drying up of semen, and infertility. Wet dreams (or 'nightfalls', as they are called in the vernacular), too, are a cause for concern among the misinformed, though they are considered normal by the medical fraternity.

Women, too, can climax in sleep after an erotic dream. Men fear that their sperm stock will diminish, resulting in infertility and impotence, and reveal these habits to the doctor in secret if the couple is infertile. Nothing can be further from the truth. Moreover, there is no such thing as a semen stock. Just as our saliva does not dry up as long as we live, no matter how much we eat, semen also does not finish for the simple reason that it is not 'stocked' but produced on a regular basis throughout life.

Health Benefits

The AMA (American Medical Association) declared masturbation normal in 1972. It is a medically and psychologically healthy habit as long as it does not become a compulsion that interferes with day-to-day activity. There is scientific evidence to prove that masturbation has beneficial effects on the physical and psychological health of an individual. These include release of sexual tension, a sense of well-being, reduced stress, relaxation, better sleep, and bolstered immunity. It can be done by people of all genders, with or without a partner. In women, it reduces menstrual pain and migraine and familiarises her with her erotic zones. Some psychiatrists believe that it helps patients with depression.

Masturbation and Partnered Individuals

Quite a few people masturbate despite the availability of a partner. Why do they feel the need to do so? One of the reasons could be that, though their partner is not sexually satisfying, they want to continue in the relationship or marriage because of love, children, or social and financial constraints, and do not want their partner to feel inadequate. One partner could be more highly sexed than the other; masturbation smoothens out the difference in libidos and promotes a harmonious relationship.

Men who suffer from premature ejaculation can masturbate the aroused woman to orgasm after the act. Mutual masturbation may be indulged in by a couple if the woman wants to preserve her virginity or by elderly couples who find it difficult to perform on account of vaginal pain or erectile dysfunction. Some women masturbate even if they have a satisfactory sex partner, for an orgasm after masturbation is often more intense than after sex.

Medical View through the Ages

In the nineteenth century, the medical fraternity thought masturbation to be a cause of insanity. Treatment varied from the mild, like eating bland, meatless meals, to the dire, like electrical shocks, to the bizarre, like chastity belts and straitjackets. Surgical treatment included circumcision, clitoral, or even genital excision. All this changed in the twentieth century when Thomas Szasz made the statement in 1973 in his book *The Second Sin*: 'Masturbation: the primary sexual activity of mankind. In the nineteenth century, it was a disease; in the twentieth, it's a cure.'

In the UK in 2009, a leaflet issued by the NHS went so far as to say, 'An orgasm a day keeps the doctor away.'

Dörner and others wrote in their now-classic book in 1978, '. . . only if I can offer something to myself can I also offer it to someone else.'

Nowadays, doctors use masturbation as a medical tool in certain situations. Sex therapists recommend that women with sexual inadequacies masturbate till orgasm to improve their sexual health and interpersonal relationships so that they can inform their partners what is erotically pleasing to them.[7] It has been encouraged in correction centres (pornographic material is supplied to inmates) to reduce the incidence of sexual assaults and rape in prison.[8] Masturbatory sperm samples are required for ART (assisted reproductive techniques) and sperm banks.[9] Men with testicular cancer can preserve their semen before radiation therapy so that they can have children later in life.

When Masturbation Becomes Abnormal

Masturbation is considered abnormal if it inhibits partner-oriented behaviour, interferes with day-to-day life, is done in public, is compulsive, or involves risky behaviour such as insertion of objects that can get stuck or cause injury. Excessive masturbation could be an indicator of sexual abuse.

Religion and Self-Gratification

The *Kama Sutra* does not condemn masturbation. In fact, it explains in detail the best way to masturbate. However, as Hinduism advocates a balanced approach to life, no aspect of living should be given more importance than another, and this holds true for masturbation, too. It is believed to lead to energy loss. Masturbation and sex began to be considered sinful when Victorian morality was thrust upon Hindus through British education during their long rule over the country.

While Hindus believed that masturbation led to energy loss, the Sumerians were of the opinion that it enhanced sexual potency and even considered it an act of creation.[10] They believed that their god Enki created the rivers Tigris and Euphrates by ejaculating into empty riverbeds after masturbation. The ancient Egyptians, too, regarded masturbation by a deity as an act of creation, for that was how the god Atum created the universe.[11] The ancient Greeks considered masturbation a healthy substitute for sex, as we do today. In the present day, Catholics, Muslims, Buddhists, and Jews forbid it, while other religions have nothing to say for or against it. Though self-gratification is rampant, those belonging to religions and cultures against masturbation end up feeling guilty without reason.

Masturbation and the Law

The prosecution of masturbation has varied at different times, from an offence punishable by death in seventeenth-century Puritan societies to total acceptance. These days, public masturbation is prosecuted in most countries under general laws of public indecency.

Strangely, there is no recognised legal category for public masturbation in the Indian Penal Code. However, it is punishable by up to fourteen days in prison in the UK, while laws vary from state to state in the US. The Supreme Court of Alabama criminalises the distribution of sex toys.

I would like to end my discussion on masturbation with an interesting piece of information I came across while researching for this chapter. A fourth-century BC cynic philosopher often masturbated in public. When scandalised people confronted him, he replied, 'If only it were as easy to banish hunger by rubbing my belly.'

How true!

6

Three in a Marriage

In the scandalous interview of Princess Diana, the veteran *Panorama* journalist Martin Bashir asked her if Camilla Parker Bowles was a factor in the breakdown of her marriage.

'Well, there were three of us in this marriage, so it was a bit crowded,' she replied.

Royal adultery indeed, but as an Indian journalist quipped, 'and then she went on to add a fourth and a fifth . . .' referring to her numerous lovers.

The word 'adultery' is derived from the Latin *adulterium* and refers to extramarital sex. The Merriam-Webster Dictionary defines adultery (or infidelity) as 'voluntary sexual intercourse between a married person and someone other than that person's current spouse or partner.' The other person in an adulterous relationship may be married or unmarried. Such an act breaches social norms, the tenets of religion, morality, and law. Besides the destruction of the family unit and the psychological impact on children and the injured partner, as well as the guilt of the erring partner, infidelity has far-reaching social, legal, and religious consequences. If it does not lead to divorce—which in itself is devastating—the fissure in the marriage remains, no matter how hard the couple tries to maintain a semblance of normalcy.

Yet, despite these repercussions, the prevalence of infidelity is about 20–25 per cent, which means that one partner in every four to five marriages has had sex with someone other than his or her spouse. Adultery is usually committed with someone known to the person, though some pay for sex outside marriage.

Society is kinder to men who have extramarital affairs. Though twice as many married men have sex outside marriage as women, a man is less forgiving of an erring wife. This is because a cuckold is the laughing stock of society on account of the prevailing belief that he was not man enough to satisfy his wife; more importantly, he might end up raising another man's child. The very word 'cuckold' comes from the cuckoo, the bird that lays its eggs in another bird's nest for it to raise. Thankfully, due to the availability of contraception and easy access to abortion, such pregnancies do not often reach term. Even if they do, paternity tests can now confirm or rule out the issue. However, many jurisdictions have set a legal time limit from a child's birth during which paternity may be challenged. Children born out of adultery suffer adverse legal and social consequences through no fault of their own. The term 'bastard' dogs them throughout life, often leading to psychological issues.

There is no way to predict how a man may react to his wife's infidelity. Reactions can range from rage to jealousy and end in separation, divorce, homicide, or suicide. There may be emotional, physical, or financial abuse if he chooses to continue the marriage for the sake of the children or to keep up social appearances. The wife and her paramour may lose their lives on account of illicit passion, or they may kill the husband (even children) to get them out of the way.

One horrific incident caught on CCTV revealed a woman who got her lover and his friend to strangle her husband. She then had sex with both of them on the adjoining bed, with her husband's body not yet cold.

If the husband does not redeem himself through honour killing, society does not spare those who dare to go against socio-religious norms. In some countries, public stoning is still the prescribed punishment for adulterers—a shameful, painful, and horrific way to die.

Wives are usually more tolerant of straying husbands. This is because most of them, at least in India, are financially, sexually, and socially dependent on their husbands and have nowhere to go. Parents, too, often refuse refuge, even if the woman is financially independent. However, there are marriages where the husband forgives his wife because he genuinely loves her, stands to gain financially, fears public disgrace, or has children to consider.

Though the repercussions of adultery are many, people do indulge in extramarital affairs even when they cannot fault their spouses. The reasons range from boredom, routine, and predictable sex to long hours spent with another person at the workplace. A young secretary, dazzled by the power and position of her employer, may allow sexual liberties that, in turn, help him tide over his midlife crisis. At times, the wife has an affair with her husband's best friend or neighbour. Those with a higher libido than their partners seek sex elsewhere, even with sex workers. An older woman may seduce a younger boy, as seen in the path-breaking film of my youth, *The Graduate*, only to learn later that he is her teenage daughter's boyfriend! Those who wish to enjoy the comforts offered by a rich husband do not break the marriage on account of poor sex; instead, they hire gigolos to satisfy their needs.

In India, where arranged marriages are still the norm, parents take into consideration caste, creed, social status, and horoscopes, but not compatibility, least of all sexual compatibility, which, all said and done, lays the foundation of a sound marriage. As a result, many go through the farce of marriage for the sake of their children, societal pressure, or financial constraints and indulge in extramarital sex to fill the void in their lives. In large joint families, it is often with brothers-in-law or even fathers-in-law, on account of proximity and lack of suspicion.

Extramarital sex exposes both the adulterer and the innocent spouse to STIs, including AIDS. Blackmail by the paramour is a very real threat, as is public exposure and punishment meted out by the injured partner, society, and the law, which can be extremely harsh. These vary according to jurisdiction. In some countries, adultery is a criminal act; in others, a civil offence that may be grounds for divorce. In jurisdictions such as Sudan, the third party is considered the offender and not the adulterous spouse. This was the case in India, too, until recently.

India's adultery law (Section 497 of the Indian Penal Code) held the man guilty, stating that the married woman was a helpless victim and free from 'criminal responsibility'. According to this law, any person who had sexual intercourse with a married woman without the consent or connivance of her husband committed the offence of adultery. The punishment could include imprisonment for up to five years, a fine, or both. The law treated women as the personal property of their husbands, which went against their basic dignity.

On 27 July 2018, the Supreme Court unanimously struck down Section 497 of the Indian Penal Code, holding that it violated:

1. Article 14 of the Constitution, which guarantees the right to equality, as it penalised only men,
2. Article 15(1), which prohibits discrimination on grounds of sex, and
3. Article 21, which protects life and personal liberty.

There is one exception, however. Despite the decriminalisation of adultery in 2018, it remains an offence in the armed forces, as it can erode trust and morale.

Adultery is now a civil offence in India and is a ground for divorce under both Hindu and Muslim personal laws. Additionally, if a Muslim woman can prove that she was falsely accused of adultery by her husband, she may sue him for divorce.

All said and done, adultery is as old as the institution of marriage. Some go so far as to claim that humans were never meant to be monogamous. Yet, as marriage remains the basic unit for raising a family, social, moral, and legal objections to adultery persist. This has not stopped people from straying, and marriages do fall apart on this account. As rationality and desire cannot coexist, the erring couple plunges headlong into dark waters, in the throes of passion made all the more powerful for being illicit. Some do find their soulmates in such liaisons, divorce their spouses, and live happily ever after—but this is not always the case. That the lives of innocent children are destroyed as collateral damage is something few consider before taking this irrevocable step.

Adultery in Literature

Being a writer myself (though not of much renown), I know that fiction is often wrapped around a core of truth, like an oyster forming a pearl around a grain of sand. I was, therefore, not surprised to learn that many famous works of literature based on extramarital affairs—Tolstoy's *Anna Karenina*, Flaubert's *Madame Bovary*, D. H. Lawrence's *Lady Chatterley's Lover*, and F. Scott Fitzgerald's *The Great Gatsby*—are loosely based on real-life stories of women who dared to breach social norms. Even Nathaniel Hawthorne found inspiration for *The Scarlet Letter* in a document he came across while working as a surveyor at the Custom House. It was enclosed in a scarlet, gold-embroidered patch of cloth in the shape of an 'A', which an adulterous woman had been forced to wear on her breast in Puritan society some two hundred years earlier.

Anna Karenina was inspired by the story of Anna Stepanovna Pirogova, the mistress of one of Tolstoy's friends, who committed suicide by jumping in front of a train. Tolstoy even observed the autopsy of the unfortunate woman.

Madame Bovary was partly inspired by the sensational case of Delphine Delamare, a French woman who left her rural home at the age of seventeen to marry a health officer who, like Dr Charles Bovary, was also a widower. In her case, sheer boredom and an inability to reconcile real life with unrealistic romantic dreams made her feel trapped in her marriage to a dull doctor who loved her in his own insipid way. Her craving for excitement and finery led her down a destructive path of debauchery, debt, and finally a horrific death by arsenic.

As for *Lady Chatterley's Lover*, D. H. Lawrence fashioned the heroine's persona on his own wife, Frieda. She was married to a German aristocrat—a professor twelve years older than her—whom she abandoned, along with her three young children, to indulge in a torrid affair with the penniless son of a coal miner (Lawrence himself), six years her junior. In those days, aristocratic women did not even speak to men of the lower classes, let alone sleep with them. He was unequal to her in every way except for sexual compatibility—something she had never enjoyed with her first husband. They married and moved abroad, away from the unforgiving eyes of England. That she later went on to have other affairs is another matter.

Even in *The Great Gatsby*, art closely imitates life. The character of Daisy Buchanan was inspired by Ginevra King, a beautiful and wealthy debutante with whom Fitzgerald fell in love when he was a poor student at Princeton. Their affair lasted two years but could not culminate in marriage, as her father told him, 'Poor boys shouldn't think of marrying rich girls.' A line that eventually found its way into the novel. When he became rich, Daisy would visit him surreptitiously but withdrew into the cocoon of her high-society life when matters got messy. Finally, Gatsby gets killed by the husband of Daisy's husband's paramour, under the mistaken notion that Gatsby was her lover!

Years later, when Fitzgerald had become famous, Ginevra met him and asked if the heroine of his novel was based on her. He reportedly replied by asking her which of the many 'bitches' he had written about she was referring to.

⚤

All said and done, adultery extracts an exacting price, be it in the form of the breakdown of a marriage or a permanent fissure in marriages that continue doggedly, plagued by a plethora of negative emotions such as lingering hurt, guilt, and mistrust. Last, but not least, is the toll it takes on children.

It is futile to warn a person venturing into forbidden territory to 'look before you leap', for in the beginning, passion clouds reason, pleasure overrides guilt, thrill speeds past caution, and consequences, however dire, are barely considered. However much they may justify their defiance or placate their conscience, they often end up burning in the fires of their private hell. As for the 'lucky' ones who divorce their spouses to marry their partner in crime, many are left with the unsettling feeling that the forbidden fruit of illicit love was far sweeter than its reality. Moreover, a lingering fear remains at the back of their minds: If one could betray a spouse for another, what guarantee is there that history will not repeat itself?

An expert once quipped, 'The trick is not to avoid an affair but to avoid getting caught.' This, however, is easier said than done, for more often than not one partner becomes emotionally dependent and wants more from the relationship, while greed prompts another to resort to blackmail; still others turn to murder or suicide as a last resort. A recent newspaper article depicted the sordid tale of a couple in their fifties who were caught indulging in an extramarital affair by the woman's twenty-eight-year-old daughter. When she threatened to inform her father, they killed her and attempted to pass it off as a 'dowry death', implicating her innocent in-laws, until the two were forced to confess under duress.

7

Exploring Same-Sex Relationships

When I visited my son in the US, he decided to take me to meet a couple of his female friends. Wondering which of the two girls would be my future daughter-in-law, I could barely contain my excitement. My son was a doctor and an eligible bachelor but showed no signs of settling down. Perhaps this was his way of telling me that he had finally decided to marry. My hopes were dashed when he told me that the two were lesbians. I am ashamed to say that I recoiled, though I managed to keep an impassive front. There was a difference between reading about homosexuality—which, as a doctor, I knew was no longer considered a disease—and being actually confronted by a pair.

I had also felt some pity for a female couple I had read about in the newspaper who died in a suicide pact, as one was being forcibly married. However, there was a difference between accepting the existence of homosexuality in a vague, distant sort of way and being in its presence personally. Here I was, on my way to visit a pair. What did I expect? Horns growing out of their heads? What did I fear? That homosexuality was contagious, and they would corrupt my son? Or was he gay himself, and this was his way of easing me into the truth of his sexuality? Was this the reason he had refused marriage proposals from eligible girls? Such were the thoughts that troubled me as we raced through the beautiful American countryside to their suburban residence.

The girls were gracious hosts; they had prepared a sumptuous meal that included a barbecue. They were happy, fun-loving women who did well in their respective jobs. I returned after a thoroughly enjoyable evening, ashamed at having judged them solely based on their sexuality. What they did in their bedroom was no concern of mine. My views changed drastically after meeting them. I thought it was daring of them to come out of the closet and hold their own in an unforgiving society.

⚤

Homosexuality denotes a romantic, emotional, and sexual attraction or behaviour between members of the same sex. The preference of a person for members of the same or opposite sex is defined as the individual's sexual orientation. This is not to be confused with sexual identity, which refers to how a person perceives himself or herself as a sexual being. A man may feel like a female trapped in a male body, while a girl may feel like a man trapped in a woman's body. After several counselling sessions, people with an identity crisis may undergo multiple surgeries and hormone therapy to change their sex and are ultimately at peace with themselves.

Along with heterosexuality and bisexuality, homosexuality is one of the three main categories of sexual orientation, though some people are asexual. Homosexuality has existed since time immemorial, with attitudes towards it varying across cultures and historical periods, ranging from a crime punishable by death to a normal, accepted way of life. Homosexual behaviour has also been noted in many animal species. In their 2016 literature review, Bailey et al. stated that they 'expect that in all cultures . . . a minority of individuals are sexually predisposed (whether exclusively or non-exclusively) to the same sex.'[12] Men are more likely to be exclusively homosexual than equally attracted to both sexes, while the opposite is true for women. Sexual orientation is stable in most cases, though at times people, usually women, may experience a change in their sexual orientation. Society often believes that if a man appears masculine, he is heterosexual, while male homosexuals are effeminate and female homosexuals appear masculine. This is not always true.

The word 'homosexual' is derived from the Greek *homos*, meaning 'same' (not the Latin *homo*, meaning 'man'). These days, the word 'gay' is commonly used for men and 'lesbian' for women attracted to members of the same sex. The word homosexual is often avoided as it connotes sexual behaviour alone, without taking into consideration the romantic or emotional attachment of the individual.

The acronym LGBTQ+ stands for lesbian, gay, bisexual, transgender, and queer people. Queer is a term used for non-normative identities or for those exploring their sexual or gender identity, while the plus sign (+) stands for intersex, asexual, pansexual, or gender-fluid identities. The word lesbian is derived from the name of the Greek island Lesbos, where Sappho (630–570 BCE), a highly esteemed poet with a sexual predilection for women, was born. From various ancient texts, it is understood that a group of young women were left in Sappho's charge for cultural edification. She wrote poetry about their lives, beauty, and her love and passion for women. Lesbians are also called 'Sapphics' after her.

Delving further into history, while sodomy between men, men and women, and men and animals was punishable by death in England, acknowledgement of sexual contact between women was non-existent in medical and legal texts. The earliest recorded execution for lesbianism occurred in Germany in 1477. Nuns who 'rode' each other or touched each other's breasts were ordered to perform penance. An Italian nun named Sister Benedetta Carlini seduced a number of other nuns while supposedly possessed by a 'Divine Spirit', for which she was placed in solitary confinement for the last forty years of her life.

In South Africa, women have been raped by heterosexual men as punishment for their 'abnormal' behaviour—an act supervised at times by members of the woman's family or the local community. Though legally South Africa protects gay rights, no proactive measures have been taken by the government to prevent 'corrective rape', which appears to be on the rise and contributes significantly to HIV infection among lesbians.

On the other hand, *motsoalle* (a very special friend) is the term for a socially acceptable, even celebrated, long-term relationship between women in Lesotho, an enclaved country surrounded by South Africa. Motsoalle relationships differ from lesbian relationships in that these women marry men and conform to gender expectations. The belief here is that an act is not considered sexual if it does not involve penile penetration; therefore, whatever these women do together is not regarded as sex, even if it involves erotic elements.

Noted Urdu writer Ismat Chughtai had to face a court trial for writing a short story titled *Lihaaf*, which hinted at the goings-on between the wife of a nawab and her maid under a quilt, while her lord was engaged in pleasurable activities elsewhere. The story was based on something she had witnessed as a child while living with an aunt. The film *Fire* was another milestone that gave greater visibility to the lesbian experience in India. After homosexuality was decriminalised by the Supreme Court, lesbians have been 'coming out' in increasing numbers.

Terms such as butch (masculine) and femme (feminine) are used in the lesbian community to organise sexual relationships and gender identity. These labels are associated with certain traits, behaviours, dress, and hairstyles, but they are not the sole form of lesbian representation, as there are many women in butch–butch and femme–femme relationships.

Cause

The exact cause of sexual orientation is not known, but it may occur due to a complex interplay of genetic, environmental, and hormonal influences. Research has found changes, called methylation patterns, in nine regions of the genome that appear to be closely linked to sexual orientation. These can predict a person's sexual orientation with an accuracy of almost 70 per cent. While religion and culture may believe that homosexuality is unnatural, there is scientific evidence to prove that it is a normal and natural variation of human sexuality. Psychological interventions do not change one's sexual orientation, for a person cannot choose to be homosexual. Parenting, early childhood experiences, and sociocultural environment do not impact it.

Earlier, homosexuality was listed as a mental disorder, but it was removed from the Diagnostic and Statistical Manual of Mental Disorders (DSM) in 1973 by the American Psychiatric Association. It is now considered a normal and positive variation of human sexual orientation and not a mental disorder that requires treatment.

The Supreme Court of India decriminalised homosexuality in 2018 (Section 377). Though it is still punishable by death in many countries, there is some laxity in the implementation of this law. Since the end of the twentieth century, there has been a global effort towards non-discrimination and equality for LGBTQ+ people in all respects, including healthcare, marriage, and adoption. Scientific research has shown that lesbian and gay parents are as fit and capable as heterosexual parents. Children raised by same-sex parents are psychologically healthy and well-adjusted and do not have a higher rate of homosexuality. Moreover, countries such as the US protect children with same-sex orientation from psychological and physical trauma due to bullying by introducing anti-bullying laws.

LGBTQ+ people deserve the dignity of a normal life in an accepting society; they have been stigmatised far too long by religious and political groups and caricatured in films and the media. This has led to homophobia and ostracisation, causing irreparable harm to people who cannot help being what they are. As it is, the LGBTQ+ group faces challenges that are not encountered by minority ethnic groups. This is because the latter usually live together in societies with a common culture and a support system in place, whereas LGBTQ+ people often live singly in communities that are ignorant, unsupportive, or openly hostile towards them. On account of prejudice and discrimination, many of them do not have the courage to come out and live a stifled life, caged in isolation, which may lead to suicide.

'Coming out of the closet' is a term used for a person who voluntarily discloses his or her sexual orientation to the world. There are three stages of 'coming out' or disclosure. First, one acknowledges one's sexual orientation to oneself—internal coming out. Secondly, one comes out to family, friends, and colleagues and finally lives openly as an LGBTQ+ person.

'Outing' is the practice of publicly revealing the sexual orientation of a closeted person by others for vested interests. Noted politicians, celebrities, members of the armed forces, and clergy have been outed with the intent of bringing about their downfall.

Health

The American Psychiatric Association 'opposes any psychiatric treatment, such as "reparative" therapy that is based upon the assumption that homosexuality is a mental disorder.' No major mental health professional organisation sanctions efforts to change sexual orientation; virtually all have cautioned the public against treatments that claim to do so. Therefore, families should not attempt to 'correct' this perceived affliction through godmen or personnel of dubious repute. Being the first point of social contact, parents should be educated to view homosexuality in the right perspective, as should teachers and social workers, so that bewildered youth know that they have support in a hostile world. It is important that they live in an open, loving environment that embraces their sexuality, allowing them to grow into healthy, well-adjusted human beings.

More often than not, the stigma associated with homosexuality leads to an increased incidence of mental health disorders such as depression, substance abuse, and suicide, owing to a hostile environment. Individuals may be subjected to verbal and physical abuse and rejection, even by members of their own family. As a result, some may run away from home or indulge in high-risk sexual behaviour with multiple partners.

Regarding physical health, as AIDS was first identified in homosexual men and continues to have a higher prevalence in this subgroup, as does hepatitis B, many countries do not allow gay men to donate blood. Lesbians are relatively safer with regard to STIs, though bisexual women may acquire infections from male partners and transmit them to female partners. STIs such as human papillomavirus (HPV) can spread between women through skin-to-skin contact, leading to warts in some cases and cervical cancer in others. Lesbians often do not visit gynaecologists as frequently as they should, as they do not require contraception or pregnancy-related consultations. Consequently, fewer Pap smears are performed, leading to delayed diagnosis of genital cancers. When medical attention is sought, sexual identity may not be disclosed for fear of a negative reaction.

However, lesbians are not exempt from infections such as trichomoniasis, bacterial vaginosis, candidiasis, herpes simplex, and syphilis; incidence depends on sexual practices. Contact with cervical secretions, vaginal mucosa, or menstrual blood through fingers or penetrative objects increases risk. Oro-genital contact exposes them to a higher risk of acquiring herpes simplex. Though less common, HIV may occur in lesbians who also have sex with men or engage in intravenous drug use. Obesity and smoking, both of which are more common among lesbians, increase the risk of heart disease.[13] Higher body mass may be related to the absence of social pressure to conform to conventional ideals of female attractiveness.

Safe sex for lesbians includes avoiding contact with a partner's menstrual blood, other body fluids, and genital lesions. Sex toys that penetrate the vagina or anus should be covered with a condom if shared between partners; ideally, each person should have a separate toy. Barriers such as condoms or dental dams should be used during oral sex. Gloves and lubricants are recommended for manual sex that may cause bleeding.

These days, the LGBTQ+ community and their supporters come out in large numbers annually in gay parades, known as Pride marches, to proclaim and celebrate their sexual orientation. The first Pride march in India—indeed, in South Asia—was held in Kolkata in 1999. It is now also held in cities such as Delhi (from 2008), Mumbai (since 2005, though on a larger scale from 2008), Hyderabad (since 2013), Chennai (2009), and Pune (2013) to promote visibility, rights, and acceptance.

While society has become more aware of sexual behaviours other than heterosexuality, it has yet to embrace them wholeheartedly. Homophobia still haunts this minority, and ridicule continues to taunt them, for there remains a wide gap between legalisation and social acceptance. Then there are the ongoing struggles for the legal recognition of same-sex marriage and adoption. In 2023, the Supreme Court ruled that it was up to Parliament to legislate on the matter, as there is no fundamental right to marry under the Constitution. As of now, queer couples can live together and receive certain benefits. Though a battle has been won, the war for equality in all respects still rages on. We can add our might by being more accepting of people whose sexual orientation does not align with ours. As they are like the rest of us, contributing to society in every way, they certainly do not deserve to be discriminated against in any way.

8

No Means No

Those who have seen the impactful film Pink understand that it revolves around the concept of consent. Three modern, sexually active girls befriend three strangers in a bar, enjoy the drinks they buy, and exchange dirty jokes with them. The boys begin to think that these girls are an easy lay and anticipate a night of debauchery. Each lures a girl into a separate room in the hotel on some pretext and begins making passes that are totally unacceptable.

This genuinely surprises the men, who have grown up believing that women who wear provocative dresses, like to have hard drinks, and exchange dirty jokes with men are 'loose'. The girls barely escape being mauled; however, the heroine ends up hitting her sexual predator on the head with a glass bottle, leaving a profusely bleeding gash. They lodge a complaint with the police and return to their shared accommodation. The wounded leader of this randy gang is the son of a politician and threatens them with dire consequences if they do not withdraw their FIR. A long-drawn court battle follows, during which the girls' reputations are torn to shreds and their consensual sexual activity with other men is exposed to public ridicule. The final take-home message, explained eloquently by their eccentric retired lawyer (played beautifully by Amitabh Bachchan), is simple: 'No means no.'

Any type of forceful sexual activity—such as kissing, fondling, oral, or genital sex—is tantamount to sexual assault. This is a crime even if the woman concerned is a prostitute, a girlfriend, a fiancée, or someone with whom consensual sex has occurred before. Forcing sex on a reluctant wife is marital rape, and it is grossly underreported.

Following the Nirbhaya gang rape case, The Criminal Law (Amendment) Act, 2013 came into force with effect from 3 February 2013, and the definition of rape after the amendment of Section 375 is as follows:

A man is said to commit 'rape' if he:

1. Penetrates his penis, to any extent, into the vagina, mouth, urethra, or anus of a woman, or makes her do so with him or any other person.
2. Inserts, to any extent, any object or a part of the body (not being the penis) into the vagina, urethra, or anus of a woman, or makes her do so with him or any other person.
3. Manipulates any part of the body of a woman so as to cause penetration into the vagina, urethra, or anus, or any part of the body of such woman, or makes her do so with him or any other person.
4. Applies his mouth to the vagina, anus, or urethra of a woman, or makes her do so with him or any other person.

Essentially, the crux of the amended rape law under Section 375 of the Indian Penal Code (IPC) is that it includes sexual activity with a woman against her will; without her consent; with consent obtained by putting her, or any person she is interested in, in fear of death or hurt; with consent given under the misconception that the man was her husband; or when consent is given by reason of unsoundness of mind, intoxication, or the influence of any stupefying or unwholesome substance. Also included are sexual acts with a woman under eighteen, with or without her consent, or with a woman who is unable to communicate consent.

This reiterates the fact that consent is of paramount importance before indulging in any sort of sexual activity with a woman. No one has the right to make a woman feel disrespected, scared, or uncomfortable during sex; it should feel good. Giving consent for one activity does not mean that a woman has given consent for a man to proceed further. For example, if she allows him to kiss her, it does not give him the right to lift her dress, go all the way, or assume permission for recurring sexual contact. In fact, even if a girl has agreed to have sex with a man but begins to feel uncomfortable midway, she is completely within her rights to back out at whatever stage of sexual activity they are in. Anything contrary to the above is against the law. However, most women do not have the courage to ask a man to stop once they have given in. They are also unable to refuse sex with a man they may have had sex with before but do not wish to now. It is important for her to know that she is within her legal rights to refuse. Consent is essential each time she engages in sexual activity, even with the same man.

It is all very well to talk about consent, but how does one go about taking consent for such a delicate issue as sex? It is not as if one is giving consent for a medical examination or a surgical operation by signing a form before allowing the doctor to proceed. A man could know that she is willing if she does not resist his advances, utters words of endearment, and responds to his kisses and hugs—provided it is not under duress or intoxication. Subtle questions such as 'Is it okay?' 'What would you like me to do?' or 'What feels good for you?' could pave the way for mutually satisfying, consensual sexual activity.

On the other hand, a woman does not necessarily have to mouth the word 'no'. Many indicators in her behaviour will let a man know that she is not comfortable with what he is doing. If she turns her face when he tries to kiss her, pulls down her dress when he is lifting it, pushes him away, or backs away from his fondling or fingering, he should stop.

Men should understand that dressing sexily, flirting, or accepting a ride or a drink does not mean consenting to anything more. Saying 'yes' (or saying nothing) out of fear, pressure, or under the influence of drugs or alcohol is not consent. Parents should teach their sons to respect *all* women. It should be impressed upon their minds that taking advantage of a woman's sexuality is not their birthright, and that women have desires and preferences of their own that need to be taken into consideration for a mutually satisfying relationship.

Rape

Can there be a more sinister four-letter word than 'rape'? It is not only a woman's body that is violated but her very soul. Not only are her private parts torn to shreds, but her self-esteem as well. Not only has she lost her honour, but also her faith in men—more so if her violator is someone she trusted and expected to protect her.

Not a single day passes without an incident of rape being reported in the newspaper, so much so that people have become blasé about it. Particularly heartrending was a tiny item about a toddler who was raped by her grown neighbour. As if this was not enough, the psychopath thrust a glass bottle into the baby's vagina and, believing her to be dead, escaped to his village. A faint mewling alerted her parents, who broke open the door to witness a scene no parent should ever see.

The gruesome Nithari serial murder case of 2006, in which the dismembered body parts of seventeen children (ten girls) were found in a drain behind the house of Moninder Singh Pandher, still sends shivers down my spine. It is said that his manservant, Surinder Koli, would kill the children by suffocating them, rape their dead bodies, cook and eat parts of their tender flesh—for example, the liver—put the bones in polythene bags, and throw them into the drain. There were rumours of organ trade and paedophilia that were never confirmed. The two were arrested and sentenced to death but, much to the dismay of the parents whose children had died such horrific deaths, were released seventeen years after conviction. A horror story of a magnitude that even the most imaginative mind could not have conceived.

The Nirbhaya gang rape case is another blot on humankind. She was raped by six men in a moving bus. The most vicious of them was a juvenile who thrust a rod into her vagina, tearing it open and bringing out tangled loops of intestine. After this, she and her boyfriend—who was injured while trying to protect her—were thrown out naked on the roadside on the cold winter night of 16 December 2012. With only five per cent of her intestines left, she survived long enough to give details of her horror. There was a nationwide uproar that brought about a significant change in the definition of rape and rape laws in India. Sadly, this has not put the fear of God into men, for the incidence of rape has not decreased. Delhi, the capital of my country, has earned the shameful title of 'the rape capital of the world'.

It is a rare Phoolan Devi who channels her angst into revenge and guns down the high-caste men who gang raped her. Speaking of the caste system, the latest unsavoury tale to join this bandwagon is that of a Dalit girl who joined a college to become a teacher. It was a first for a girl of her caste in her village, and she became a role model for others. The high castes were unable to tolerate her presence in the college hostel and made her do menial tasks. Time and again, she was sent to clean the room and toilet of a male teacher who raped her with impunity. Her body was eventually found in the college water tank. Because of the public outcry, this became one of those rare cases in which a high-caste man was arrested. Usually, they roam free with the connivance of the police. What I fail to understand is that, though discrimination between castes is such that a lower caste person cannot even drink water from a 'high-caste' well, how do these high-caste men bring themselves to touch an 'untouchable' girl, let alone perform such an intimate act with her? If the hapless lower-caste girl dares to seek justice, she is hounded and harassed until she ends her life. In one case, an entire family was set ablaze at night, as they slept in their hut, because they dared to lodge a complaint against their daughter's high-caste rapists. No wonder most of them meekly tolerate such atrocities.

Of all the crimes committed against women, sexual violation is the most heinous. The culprit is often known to the girl, usually someone she trusts—father, brother, uncle, cousin, teacher, or neighbour.

Sexual intercourse with one's own wife, if she is less than 18 years old, legally amounts to rape. This is rampant in certain states where child marriage is the custom, despite laws against it. Enticing minor girls with the promise of marriage, arranging mock marriages, or keeping her as the second wife are but ploys to obtain her consent for sexual activity. Quite often, these girls (who have run away from home under the romantic influence of these crooks) are left in the lurch. Some conceive and opt for criminal abortions or suicide; others are sold to brothels. Girls in some Southern parts of India are offered as Devdasis to the goddess Yellama but end up appeasing the sexual desire of 'pious' priests. At other places, they are auctioned like cattle.

Sexual crimes against women could take the form of:

1. Molestation, when the actual act of sex does not take place, but other forms of sexual harassment are resorted to.
2. Rape, when intercourse occurs using force or threat of force.
3. Sexual intercourse with a minor, even with her consent, amounts to statutory rape.
4. Incest, when the act is committed between consanguineous (blood relatives), like sister and brother, daughter and father, or those related by lineage, like an aunt's husband. Sadly, the act is usually committed by a person with whom the girl has to remain in continual proximity. Most of the time, the mother knows that the father is violating their daughter, but keeps her mouth shut out of shame or because he is the sole earning member of the family. Usually, the perpetrator has been sexually abused himself in childhood; however, that is no excuse.
5. Sexual perversion, like exhibitionism, is when a man resorts to indecent exposure. I remember a manservant who enticed little girls to his room on the pretext of showing them a trapped bird. Instead, he unzipped his pants! Horror-struck, the girls ran away and thankfully reported the matter to their parents.

6. Paedophilia, when a grown-up man has sex with a minor of either sex.

The violation of a woman's body and trust has far-reaching physical and psychological consequences. The more trusted her assailant, the greater is her trauma. A movie based on a true incident depicts the heart-rending tale of a motherless village girl who has her first period. Her father sends her to town so that her aunt can educate her on feminine issues that are beyond him. Her aunt's husband buys ice cream and toys for the poor 12-year-old and proceeds to rapes her at this vulnerable time. The bubbly child returns to the village, a hollow shell of her original self and starts wetting her bed. Though she eventually marries her childhood sweetheart, their sex life is riddled with problems—all because of the dastardly act of an uncle she trusted.

Then there was this recent high-profile case of a 31-year-old doctor in Kolkata who was brutalised, raped, and murdered in a barbaric manner. Though this, too, led to protests, sadly, nothing has changed since the Nirbhaya case.

A woman's reaction to rape can be divided into two phases.

The acute phase, which can be overt, is when the symptoms of stress are manifested in the form of fear, weeping, tenseness, trembling, and restlessness. There could be shock, disbelief, or quiescence. The latter responses reflect avoidance reactions or coping mechanisms that require control of emotions. Emotional disturbances, such as anger, humiliation, and self-blame, or a combination of the above. At times, the reaction is controlled, when the girl's true feelings are masked under seemingly unrelated complaints like headaches, sleep disturbances, nightmares, and urinary/bowel complaints. Symptoms of acute stress disorder could be present for three days to one month after the assault.

The second phase occurs when the woman tries to come to terms with the situation but has long-range effects that include post-traumatic stress disorder (PTSD). They may re-experience the trauma in the form of flashbacks, upsetting thoughts/images, persistent blame of self, and an inability to experience positive emotions. There could be sleep difficulties, nightmares, irritability, concentration issues, phobias, and sex-related problems later in life. Evidence indicates that rape is also related to long-term physical health problems like asthma, irritable bowel syndrome, headaches, pelvic pain, or pain during intercourse.

Though the raped girl and her family are reluctant to go to the police for fear of disgrace and ruination of her marital prospects, it is wise to consult a gynaecologist because the repercussions of rape are both physical and psychological. A gynaecologist will look for genital and/or extragenital injuries that need repair and antibiotics, decrease the chances of a pregnancy and sexually transmitted diseases like HIV, Hepatitis, HPV, syphilis, gonorrhoea, chlamydia, trichomonas, candidiasis, bacterial vaginosis by prescribing medication.

Additionally, it is wise to go to the doctor/police immediately after the incident without a bath or change of clothes. Marks of injury are noted, clothes are kept as evidence, as are nail cuttings, pubic hair, blood samples, swabs from her mouth, vagina, etc. There is a prescribed protocol to be followed by the medical examiner while examining a rape victim. It is also her duty to report a case of rape, more so if the female is a minor. Whether you want to pursue a criminal case against the offender is your prerogative.

⚤

Women who reject the advances of the opposite sex fare no better. They are stalked, threatened, and have acid thrown on them, which scars their faces and psyches for life. There are incidents of the murder of girls who reject the advances of unsuitable suitors, for such men believe that 'if she cannot belong to me, she will belong to no one else'.

People tend to say that men who hound, hurt, and ravage women are worse than beasts. This is an insult to the animal kingdom, for beasts would never impose themselves on an unwilling female. They may fight amongst themselves to win her favours . . . that, too, only when she is in heat.

The world would be a better place if boys were conditioned to respect women from childhood. Till we reach this utopian state, we must protect the girl child. She should be taught the difference between a good touch and a bad touch as soon as she is old enough to understand and asked to confide in her mother regarding untoward behaviour by any male member, within the family or outside it. If she feels romantically towards a man, she should not give in to him to 'prove her love for him'. It is an age-old ploy employed by men to lure her into having sex with them. This could lead to exploitation, blackmail, and desertion—or worse still, she could end up in a brothel.

I would not like to end this discourse by making men the sole culprits. Many have been victims of violence and sexual abuse themselves in childhood. In the film *The Anatomy of Violence*, based on the 2012 Delhi gang rape, Deepa Mehta uncovers the brutalities faced by these men in their youth, which made them immune to the suffering of their victim; some even believed that she deserved it. This makes one realise that even the male child should be protected from abuse—sexual or otherwise—for his own sake and for the women he might rape later in life out of misplaced vengeance. Global research estimates that around 15 per cent of men experienced sexual violence before eighteen, and many survivors delay or never disclose their trauma due to stigma, shame, or fear.[14] This leads to psychological problems, including a tendency towards violence, later in life.

Then there are adult women who consensually indulge in premarital sex, adultery, or prostitution but cry rape when they are caught. During my second year of MBBS, I came across an interesting case in our forensic test book: A woman, who was indulging in consensual sex, shouted 'rape' on being caught in the act. An orange pip saved the man. One was found stuck between his teeth (he had eaten an orange just before sex) and another in her vagina, for he had also gone down on her.

At times, men become victims of women-friendly laws that women cunningly use against them, and families are harassed and convicted for false dowry cases. But by and large, such cases are the exception, for statistics show that violation of a woman's body occurs with alarming frequency.

Voh subah kabhi toh aayegi [there will soon come a day], when women, who are worshipped as goddesses in temples, are given the respect and dignity they deserve in real life.

9

Cosmetic Gynaecology

With gritted teeth and an unresponsive body, Rashmi waited for the mindless pounding to stop. Finally, Ranjan came and rolled over, frustrated with the joyless union. Both lay quiet in their private hells, facing away from each other; a far cry from the initial years of their marriage when they would sleep, replete in each other's arms.

Rashmi was no longer the soft, sweet-smelling woman that Ranjan had married. Under his expert guidance, the shy virgin had become a wildcat in bed, and both had looked forward to their nightly escapades. All that was before their son was born. He was one year old now, time enough for her to have healed down there, but contrary to his expectations, matters had not improved. She was still loose and there was a faint smell of urine about her. Unreasonably, he was angry with her for not being the woman he had married. He was angry with himself, too, for his dependency on her. A healthy libido needed release, but the act had now become a chore that gave no pleasure.

On her part, Rashmi felt cheated. She had suffered the agonies of childbirth to give him the child he wanted. The baby had literally ripped her apart to enter this world. The family was pleased that she had a normal birth in an era where caesareans had become the norm. In retrospect, she wondered if an operative delivery would have spared her vagina the trauma of childbirth. Their son was the joy of their lives, but the miracle of motherhood had destroyed the pleasures of wifehood.

Their unions were now a torture to be borne. They were drifting apart, and it was but a matter of time before he would seek solace elsewhere. She felt unloved and undesirable, and there was no one she could confide in, regarding a matter as intimate as this.

Miraculously, help came from unexpected quarters—Dr Anita, a cousin and gynaecologist, had just finished a course and was excited about testing her skills. She had also bought some expensive-looking equipment that she was going to use to revolutionise gynaecological practice.

'*Aisa kya kamaal karne waale ho aap* [What remarkable feat are you going to accomplish]?' asked Rashmi, not particularly interested.

'Well, I've got a certificate in Cosmetic Gynaecology, a speciality that will restore the joys of sex to thousands of women who suffer in silence; that, too, without surgery!'

Anita Didi was a godsend who had literally landed at her doorstep. One thing led to another, and—without her husband's knowledge—Rashmi became her first patient. To her utter surprise, after a few sessions, her vagina had tightened, and the embarrassing leak of urine she experienced on coughing and sneezing had disappeared.

Ranjan was in for a surprise on their wedding anniversary. She wore an alluring nightie, sprinkled fragrant jasmine on satin bedsheets, and took the initiative in bed! Needless to say, their marriage was salvaged and joy returned to their lives.

⚥

A lucrative branch of gynaecology has surfaced in recent times—cosmetic gynaecology. It has become one of the fastest-growing branches of surgery, opening up possibilities that were unheard of. As with plastic surgery elsewhere, this can be divided into reparative—when tissues damaged by the trauma of difficult childbirth or injury are repaired—and beautification. However, unlike plastic surgery, it addresses another issue, which is enhanced sexual satisfaction.

Beautification of the External Genitalia

As with other parts of the body, aesthetics is largely about an individual's own perception of beauty. Though there is no set standard of beauty regarding the external genitalia (the vulva), whatever makes one unhappy can be corrected. This often leads to an improvement in emotional well-being and one's sense of self as a sexual partner. Some may want to enhance or reduce the fat on the mons pubis, others may wish to plump up the labia majora or reduce their thickness for a sleeker look. Yet others opt for labiaplasty of the labia minora (the inner lips of the vulva) if they protrude beyond the labia majora (the outer lips). Aesthetics may not be the only reason for this, as protruding folds of skin can cause discomfort by chafing against tight clothing or interfering with intercourse.

Hymenoplasty

There is an increasing number of young women who indulge in premarital sex but, in hymen-obsessed societies like ours, wish to enter the bridal chamber of an arranged marriage with their 'virginity' restored. This can be achieved through a procedure called revirgination or hymenoplasty.

Clitoral Hood Reduction

Clitoral hood reduction is a form of female genital cosmetic surgery (FGCS) that removes excess skin over the clitoris to improve its appearance and, in some cases, enhance sexual pleasure. As most of the above-mentioned procedures are performed surgically, it is important to consult a trained specialist for adequate counselling and management.

Stress Incontinence and Vaginal Laxity

Some women develop an embarrassing condition after childbirth or menopause—urinary leakage while coughing, sneezing, or laughing. This is termed stress incontinence in medical parlance. If severe, it can consign them to a life of smelly solitude and quiet misery. Most do not seek help, believing this to be the price women pay for childbirth or menopause. Those who do consult a doctor are often offered surgery, which frightens them away.

There are also women whose vagina becomes lax after childbirth, making sex less enjoyable, particularly for their partners. Until recently, they were advised cumbersome Kegel exercises, for which they often had neither the time nor the inclination while caring for a newborn. Though the Kegella chair is a recent addition in some hospitals and helps women contract and relax their pelvic floor muscles, who has the time? Surgical tightening remained the only other option until now. With the advent of laser, radiofrequency (RF), and platelet-rich plasma (PRP), these women now need only a few OPD sittings to address their problems.

Laser Therapy

It hydrates the vaginal mucosa and regenerates collagen fibres, allowing the vagina to regain its suppleness. Collagen fibres also contract and thicken, leading to tissue shrinkage, which tightens the vagina and relieves symptoms of stress incontinence. This rejuvenation process also addresses the atrophy that sets in after menopause.

Radiofrequency (RF)

Radiofrequency vaginal rejuvenation repairs vaginal tissue by boosting collagen and elastin production and is considered superior to laser therapy. It is a quick, painless outpatient procedure that delivers controlled heat, raising the temperature of deeper tissue layers to an optimal 40–45°C, thereby triggering the production of new collagen and elastin. Unlike lasers, which burn tissue to force regeneration, RF does not damage tissue. It uses electromagnetic waves to rejuvenate and tighten the vagina while increasing elasticity and moisture. Results are almost immediate due to the formation of thicker, shorter collagen fibres. Increased blood flow to the vagina improves sexual function by reducing dryness and atrophy. Tightening of the tissue beneath the anterior vaginal wall also helps treat stress urinary incontinence.

Though treatment protocols vary depending on the degree of laxity and urinary leakage, usually three to four sessions of 15–20 minutes each, spaced four to six weeks apart, are sufficient to restore bladder control, vaginal tightness, and sexual pleasure. Sexual intercourse should be avoided for 24–48 hours after each sitting. The procedure is generally well tolerated, though mild irritation or redness may occur and resolves quickly.

Platelet-Rich Plasma (PRP)

PRP, obtained from the patient's own blood, contains various growth factors and is gaining prominence as a non-surgical treatment for female sexual dysfunction, poor lubrication, and stress urinary incontinence. It is injected beneath the vaginal skin. Being autologous, it has no known side effects. A combination of PRP and RF is a promising development in this field.

G-Spot Augmentation/Amplification

Though not universally accepted, the G-spot is described as an erotic area on the anterior vaginal wall, approximately 1–2 inches above the opening. Women keen on enhancing sexual pleasure sometimes opt for G-spot augmentation using autologous fat or PRP. Thanks to widespread propaganda, more women are becoming obsessed with various other so-called trigger spots and seek enhancement, despite the absence of robust scientific evidence supporting their existence or the efficacy of such treatments. Therefore, if one achieves climax through clitoral stimulation and enjoys a generally satisfactory sex life, one should think twice before undergoing these procedures. However, a select few women who have lost vaginal orgasmic pleasure following childbirth trauma or anterior vaginal wall surgery—leading to diminished sensation in that area—may benefit from G-spot amplification.

Vulvar Lightening

Embarrassed by hyperpigmentation of the vulva, some women opt for vulvar lightening. This involves the use of chemical agents or fractional carbon dioxide laser treatment.

Cosmetic Surgery in Adolescents

At times, young girls seek genital surgeries such as labiaplasty because they are unhappy with their appearance and worry it may displease future sexual partners. Others experience practical difficulties, as protruding labia minora can rub against tight clothing or interfere with physical activities. In such cases, parents must be involved and counselled alongside the adolescent. It is important to understand that developmental changes continue to occur in the vulva, and it is prudent to delay treatment until genital, mental, and psychological maturity has been achieved.

All said and done, the potential of cosmetic surgery is immense. It has opened up possibilities that were unheard of a generation ago and has addressed issues long considered taboo. However, before rushing into any aesthetic procedure, one must carefully deliberate its pros and cons. Consult an expert who can provide guidance on safety and long-term benefits. After all, as with any surgical intervention, there are potential risks and unintended consequences.

Part II

Sexuality through Different Phases of Life

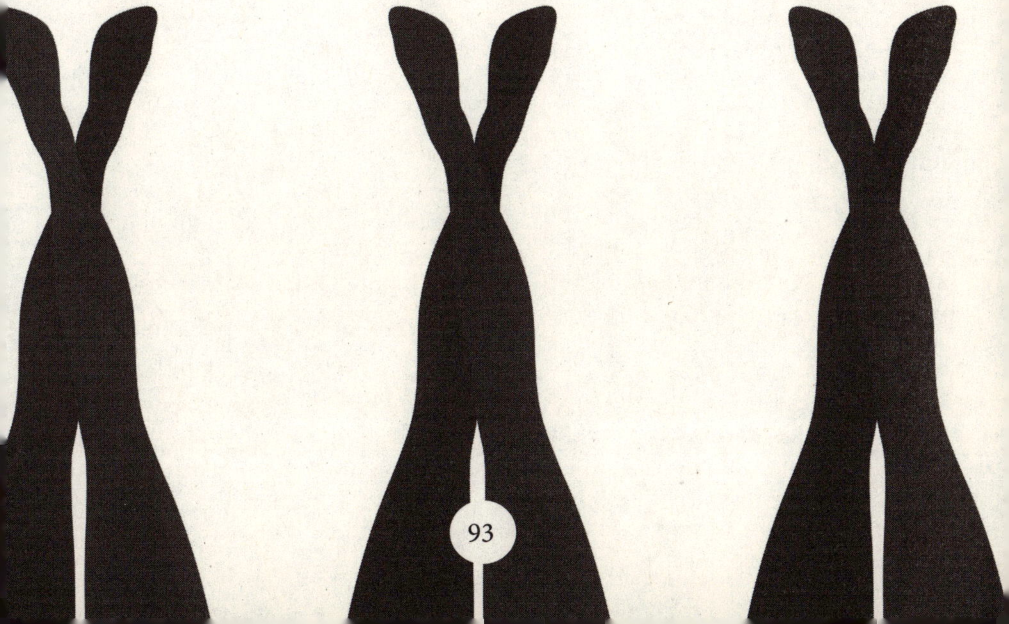

10

Understanding Childhood Sexuality

Childhood sexuality is something most of us would like to believe does not exist. In reality, young children explore their bodies, including genitals, as part of normal sensory and emotional development. When adults react with embarrassment, scolding, or punishment, they attach shame and guilt to behaviour that is normal.

From infancy, some children engage in repetitive movements or body-focused behaviours that provide pleasure and comfort. These actions can occur during everyday activities such as sitting, eating, or playing and are usually not accompanied by distress or awareness of social boundaries. As children grow, they may discover diverse ways of calming themselves, much like thumb-sucking or rocking.

In the case of one child in my family, self-stimulatory behaviour was observed from early toddlerhood. This took the form of repetitive forward and backward body movements against a full diaper or the middle strap of her pram, which provided pleasure. When these movements were abruptly interrupted, the child became distressed.

As the child grew older, the behaviour persisted in different forms, often occurring without awareness of social context or the need for privacy. Such behaviour, in an otherwise healthy child of three, caused embarrassment to her parents who did not know how to respond.

Following professional consultation, the parents were advised not to respond with punishment or shame. Instead, they were encouraged to use gentle distraction and redirection through play, outdoor activity, or interaction with other children—and to introduce concepts of privacy gradually. Clinical guidance suggests that disciplinary responses may reinforce secrecy and anxiety rather than reduce the behaviour.

In most cases, such self-stimulatory behaviours diminish naturally with age. However, persistent, compulsive, or injurious behaviours fall outside the range of typical development and warrant medical and psychological evaluation. Understanding childhood sexuality through the lens of developmental stages allows caregivers and professionals to distinguish between age-appropriate behaviour and situations that require intervention.

A mother once brought her seven-year-old son with his swollen penis stuck in a small glass bottle. Needless to say, I sent him to a surgeon to do the needful. The child would need psychological help, too. This brings us to the question of childhood sexuality through the perspective of a child's sexual development.

Sexual Development

A child's sexual development is as important as their physical, mental, and emotional growth. This begins earlier than one would expect and manifests in a variety of sexual behaviours.

Freud's phases of sexual development begin with the oral phase, which lasts until one year of age. The child derives pleasure from sucking, chewing, and eating. Then comes the anal phase between one and three years, which revolves around bowel movements and includes toilet training. Depending on how strict or lenient parents are, a child may develop an anal-retentive personality—characterised by discipline, orderliness, cleanliness, and control, possibly stemming from fear of failure during rigorous toilet training—or an anal-expulsive personality, characterised by disorderliness, lack of discipline, impulsiveness, or defiance associated with lenient or neglectful training.

This is followed by the phallic phase, which lasts between three and six years, when the child enjoys touching their genitals and is curious about the genitalia of the opposite sex.

It is followed by the latency phase, from about six years of age until puberty, when social interests engage the child and sexuality takes a back seat.

Finally comes the genital phase from puberty onwards, when sexual interest in others develops. However, modern psychologists believe that sexual development cannot be compartmentalised rigidly, as there is considerable overlap and the process is more complex than Freud believed. Much depends on genetics, environment, and the sociocultural milieu. Their own upbringing and sociocultural environment largely shape adult reactions to childhood sexuality.

A baby's earliest attachment is with the mother through physical contact. While being held, kissed, hugged, and cuddled, babies experience comforting, positive physical sensations that they learn to associate with being loved. This lays the foundation for mature physical and sexual intimacy later in life. As they grow older, children like to explore their bodies and touch their genitals.

Children enjoy being naked, like my incorrigible three-year-old twin granddaughters, who run amok in their birthday suits before and after a bath while their harried mother runs after them, frocks in hand. On the other hand, their seven-year-old brother tries hard to hide his genitals from their inquisitive eyes. They are thrilled when they do manage to catch a glimpse. Parental reactions to such behaviour give children their first lessons in sexuality.

By the age of two or three, a child begins to develop a sense of being male or female. Culture and environment teach them behavioural differences between boys and girls. Parents should decide what message they want to convey about femininity or masculinity, as gender roles are becoming increasingly blurred in changing times. Be mindful of your behaviour with the opposite sex, for children see and learn.

Between the ages of three and five, gender identity becomes more solidified, and children explore their bodies even more. Do not scold them, as this may lead to feelings of guilt and shame. Instead, explain that although such activity may give pleasure, it is not to be done in public. This is also a good time to tell them that no one else should touch them there—or anywhere—in a way that makes them feel uncomfortable.

At this stage, children may also play 'doctor-doctor', stripping in front of one another to examine and touch each other's private parts. If you catch them doing so, do not overreact; simply ask them to dress and distract them. If, however, an older child or an adult is 'doctoring' your child, this must be strictly forbidden. Preschoolers also ask many questions, such as 'Why is my brother different down there?' or 'Where do babies come from?' These should be answered in a simple, age-appropriate manner.

Between the ages of six and ten, children usually play with their peers of the same sex. This is also the age when social media begins to influence sexual attitudes, particularly if parents have not taken the initiative to teach basic facts of life. Children may be curious and giggly about mating birds and dogs. This is the time to explain that sexuality is a natural part of life, but sex is something that should be engaged in at an appropriate age and with the right person.

As the exciting yet daunting changes of puberty begin, children need parental support more than ever. They may be filled with anticipation and apprehension, and it is the duty of parents and school-based sex educators to prepare them for the physical changes that will occur. Those who mature earlier or later than their peers require special attention. The pubertal girl or boy will be more curious than ever about their body, babies, love, and sex, and these questions must be answered openly to foster a healthy sense of self-acceptance.

As girls typically begin menstruating approximately two years after breast development, they should be informed about it before their first period. Boys should also be told about menstruation so that they are sympathetic to their sisters and female classmates, rather than shaming them if they notice a bloodstain on their clothes. This is also the time to provide a more detailed explanation of how babies are conceived. If you feel emotionally unequipped to guide them through this phase, provide appropriate reading material or consult an expert.

Now that we understand the sexual development of a child, we must learn ways to differentiate normal sexual behaviour from abnormal behaviour. According to guidelines from the American Academy of Paediatrics (AAP), here's how to recognise normal and abnormal behaviour.

Normal Behaviour

They may include occasional genital touching in public or private, curiosity about bodily differences, brief attempts to look at others' bodies, or showing one's genitals to peers. These behaviours are usually transient, exploratory, and easily redirected without distress.

Less common behaviours include brief physical closeness, imitative kissing, or touching others' bodies. The latter may occur but should be infrequent, non-coercive, and responsive to clear boundaries and distraction.

Behaviours that are persistent, intrusive, resistant to redirection, or involve insertion of objects, contact with animals, or adult sexual behaviours fall outside the range of typical development and require further evaluation.

Caregivers should respond calmly, avoid shaming, redirect the child to appropriate activities, and clearly teach concepts of bodily autonomy and consent, including that no one should touch another person's private parts and that they have the right to refuse such contact themselves.

Children will ask many questions that must be answered in an age-appropriate manner. It's best not to convey embarrassment or anger through words or expressions, as this may make the child feel ashamed of their curiosity. Answer only the specific question asked, without unnecessary details.

If a preschooler asks, 'Where do babies come from?' do not say, 'We got you from the hospital' or 'The stork brought you,' as you will lose credibility when they eventually learn the truth. A simple explanation like, 'When a man and woman marry and live together, the mother's tummy grows, and the baby comes out,' is sufficient. Exposure to sexual content on social media and other platforms should be avoided. Ensure that any sexual activity in the home is conducted away from children's inquisitive eyes, lest they attempt to imitate what they observe.

Abnormal Behaviour

Some sexual behaviours are not typical and may indicate a more serious concern. These include persistent sexual behaviour from which the child cannot be distracted—sexual acts involving children more than four years apart in age, behaviour that causes emotional or physical pain or injury to self or others, use of force, simulation of adult sexual acts, or engagement in a variety of sexual behaviours daily.

The cause may range from boredom to exposure to sexually explicit material online or a personal experience of sexual abuse. Such children require professional help, which should be sought at the earliest. This does not necessarily reflect poorly on the parents, and guilt serves no purpose. Seeking help simply means prioritising the child's well-being.

A detailed history is usually be taken to assess factors such as adults moving about naked in the child's presence, lack of privacy during adult sexual activity witnessed by the child, or experiences of sexual, physical, or emotional abuse or neglect. Sudden life changes, such as the arrival of a new sibling or admission to daycare, may also contribute. Most children eventually outgrow such aberrant behaviour with appropriate intervention.

Good Touch and Bad Touch

Nothing justifies child abuse—sexual or otherwise. It is never too early to start, but it is best to do so between the ages of three and five. Begin by teaching the child proper names for all body parts, including private parts, as making up names conveys the idea that there is something shameful about the proper name.

Lessons in modesty should begin when children of a certain age like to roam about naked. Do not force children to hug or kiss people they do not want to, including grandparents. After reassuring them that most touches are okay, explain the difference between a 'good touch' and a 'bad touch'. Simply speaking, a bad touch is something you don't like and want it to stop right away.

You can explain by mentioning that the areas covered by a swimsuit are particularly sacrosanct and are not to be violated in any way. They should be taught to say 'no' to a touch that scares or confuses them. Being stripped, hit, kicked, or made to watch the exposed private parts of an adult is also not okay. Assure them that you are always there to protect them, and they must report such occurrences to you or another trusted adult immediately.

Good times to talk to your children about such things are during bath time, at bedtime, and before any new situation, especially if they have to stay back after school for dance or sports activities or are going to a camp.

At times, they may feel guilty or, in some way, responsible for the wrong done to them, which makes them reluctant to confide in anyone. At other times, they may be threatened by the perpetrator to keep quiet. In such situations, personality changes may occur, which can help alert the parents that something is amiss. For instance, if a cheery, bubbly child suddenly becomes withdrawn or morose, it is time to take note and act.

I once read a heart-rending story of two sisters in a newspaper, aged eight and six, who had run away from home but had nowhere to go. Their mother had left them in the care of a drunk father who would do bad and painful things to them. That night, they had locked themselves in the bathroom, only to learn from the screams emanating from the bedroom that he had caught hold of their five-year-old brother and was doing something awful to him. Unable to bear it any longer, they escaped through the bathroom window.

No child should ever have to suffer abuse, as the scars inflicted in childhood mark a person for life. Most adult adjustment issues—sexual or social—stem from childhood injuries, whether physical or psychological. It is our duty to nurture them in a safe and loving environment so that they grow up into healthy, well-adjusted adults.

11

An Exploration of Adolescent Sexuality

Myra was a bubbly girl in her teens. She had suddenly gained height and developed womanly curves, though the innocent smile on her pretty face remained the same. She did well in school, was kind and considerate, and had a multitude of friends with whom she chatted regularly on the mobile phone she had received on her fifteenth birthday. She had a healthy appetite, a keen mind, and a loving heart. Her parents felt blessed that Myra had not turned into the rebellious adolescent they had feared.

Suddenly, everything changed. She attended a friend's birthday party and was never the same again. Before leaving, she twirled happily in front of her mother, fishing for compliments. She did indeed look beautiful in her sunflower-yellow dress, the bodice outlining her bosom, her blow-dried hair framing her lovely face.

Someday she was going to make some man very happy, thought her mother with pride, little realising that Myra would be doing just that tonight.

A niggling fear turned to alarm when she neither answered her phone nor returned till 11 p.m. When she finally came home, humming a peppy number, her mother said, 'The least you could have done was ring up to tell us you were getting late. I was so worried . . .'

'I didn't realise it was this late. We were having such a good time.' How good a time, she dared not tell.

'And here your father and I were so worried, what with accidents . . .'

'That could happen *after* I rang up,' she retorted cheekily.

She *was* turning into an insolent teenager after all.

'Myra!' exclaimed her mother. 'You will know the torture I've gone through when you become a mother yourself!'

'Spare me the sermon, Ma,' said Myra rudely, banging the door in her face. Motherhood was the last thing on her mind. She was hugging a delicious secret to herself. With her looks and body, Myra was keen on becoming a top-class model and had taken the first step today. Being acclaimed academicians in a prestigious college, her parents would not understand. Perhaps they would appreciate her talent once she flaunted a contract with a big brand, as she had been promised. Till then, she would say nothing.

Over the next few weeks, a drastic change came over Myra. She became morose and withdrawn, her grades fell, and she startled whenever her phone rang. Her mother once found her staring blankly at the wall while her phone rang shrilly.

'Why aren't you picking up your phone?'

'I don't want to.'

'Why?'

'Shelly was mean to me in school today. I don't want to talk to her.'

'Maybe she's ringing to apologise. There is something called forgiveness,' said her mother, smiling inwardly at the irony of the situation, for most mothers wanted their offspring off the phone.

'You keep out of it, Ma,' snapped Myra angrily.

As the days passed, Myra withdrew into a shell of silence. Then the worst thing that could occur took place. Myra would not come out of her room for dinner. After calling out to her three or four times, her mother decided to let her go to bed hungry for once. She had been too soft with Myra, which made her think she could get away with anything.

But mothers are mothers after all. Before turning in for the night, Madhuri knocked at Myra's door. Not a sound emanated from her room. When repeated knocks did not elicit the now-usual 'go away' or 'leave me alone', Madhuri feared the worst. Alarmed, she called her husband, who opened the lock to Myra's door with a spare key. To their shock, they found her lying unconscious on the bed, an empty bottle of sleeping pills by her side.

Though the doctors were able to save her life, the girl who returned from the hospital was not their vivacious and animated Myra, but a broken doll with dead eyes. Life had been leached out of her very existence. In bits and pieces, her sordid story tumbled out.

She had been in talks with a modelling agency and was called for a photoshoot. That was where she had gone, on the day she pretended to attend a birthday party. The handsome photographer won her over with his sophistication and promises of great things to come, 'if only she would show a little more of her body, and then some more . . .' he cajoled as he clicked away furiously. He would breathily request a change of pose in her ear, flutter his lips fleetingly across the nape of her neck, and 'accidentally' graze his hand across her breast, showering her with lavish praise all the while. He slipped the elastic neckline of her garment over her shoulders to reveal the cleavage between the young swell of her breasts.

Overwhelmed by the onslaught of erotic stimuli, she was unbearably aroused; so was he, as she could see by the bulge in his pants. The man did not go all the way—sex, even with a consenting underage girl, would be rape, and a ruptured hymen would be proof—but he did perform oral sex until she experienced a mind-blowing orgasm, the first of her life. Promising eternal love and a brilliant career in modelling, he dropped her home.

She was happier than ever, unaware that their 'beautiful act of love' had been recorded for posterity. All too soon, she received graphic videos along with threats of exposure if she did not pay up. Myra was reduced to stealing from her trusting parents, but the blackmailer's greed kept increasing till she had no option left but to take this final step.

To cut a long story short, the cybercrime department was alerted, and the criminal was put behind bars. He confessed to luring several gullible girls in a similar manner.

Getting Myra back on track was a different matter altogether, but she had the resilience of youth and unstinting parental support. That her father had the finances to hire the best psychiatrist in town helped. Eventually, she was able put this traumatic experience behind her and move on.

⚤

Not all girls are that lucky. Most do not recover from the repercussions of their folly. The only option left for them is suicide or a life of sexual slavery. This brings to my mind the hard-hitting book, *13 Reasons Why*, now also a Netflix series about a girl called Hannah Baker who is bullied sexually—her body part exploited—has her private pictures taken surreptitiously, her innocent moves in the exciting new world of sexuality blown out of proportions so that she ends up being called the 'school slut'. Raped by the rich, school basketball star and let down by all, including her school counsellor, she takes her own life.

In the guise of relatives, classmates, neighbours, teachers, even brothers and fathers, predators lurk everywhere, and the vulnerable teenager with her burgeoning sexuality is easy prey. It is imperative that we provide young people with a secure, non-judgemental family support system and equip them with sound education in reproductive health, with special emphasis on the repercussions of high-risk sexual behaviour.

Until barely a generation ago, the bewildering changes that took place in a girl's life were kept under wraps. Menstruation came as a shock and was spoken of in hushed tones. The distraught girl was told only that she had 'become a woman' and must now be wary of men, which scared and confounded her. Sex education was unheard of in those days. Erratic and often erroneous information from equally ignorant peers perplexed her still further.

Today, the scenario represents the other extreme—equally dismal. The modern girl knows everything or believes she does. 'Information' pours in from social media, television, films, advertising, and pornography. Many believe it is fashionable to engage in premarital sex yet remain unaware of the consequences of unprotected or high-risk sexual behaviour. Parents are reluctant to discuss sex with their children, while schools often restrict sex education to the anatomy of the male and female reproductive systems and menstruation, wary of imparting the knowledge that truly matters. What adolescents require is a realistic, scientific approach to the seemingly unreal changes in their lives. Half-baked truths from questionable sources can cause irreparable harm.

Adolescence, as we know, is a period of sexual maturation. The surge of female sex hormones alters the physical contours of a child into those of a woman, preparing her body for reproduction. As sexuality is intrinsic to reproduction, profound psychosexual changes follow. Like a river in spate, her sexuality becomes a force to reckon with. A bewildering array of emotions assails her: She is excited and apprehensive, thrilled and terrified, liberated yet constrained. She welcomes her newfound sexuality, takes pride in her developing body, and is stirred by unfamiliar physical sensations. She becomes deeply invested in her appearance and is conscious of the attention she attracts. Parental authority is resented as she seeks to assert her independence. Peers take precedence over elders. This is the most vulnerable period of her life, when she can easily fall prey to substance use and sexual exploitation.

The paradox of adolescence is that sexual maturity precedes mental, emotional, and financial maturity. Delays in marriage—whether due to higher education or career aspirations—contribute to delays in socially sanctioned sexual relationships. As a result, the torrent of desire unleashed by hormonal changes may lead to high-risk sexual behaviour. The fallout can range from sexually transmitted infections (STIs), including HIV, to unintended pregnancies and unsafe abortions, which may compromise reproductive health before adulthood has truly begun.

Sexual behaviour in adolescence is influenced by education, religion, socioeconomic status, ethnicity, culture, tradition, family values, and background. Mass media, peer groups, and the presence or absence of comprehensive sex education also play a significant role. Broadly, the options available to an adolescent in navigating her sexuality include:

1. **Premarital Sex**

   Children living on the streets may engage in 'survival sex', exchanging sexual activity for food, money, protection, or substances. A significant proportion of individuals involved in sex work are adolescents. Apart from STIs, unintended pregnancies and unsafe abortions, early sexual debut and multiple sexual partners increase the risk of cervical cancer. Some girls are victims of sexual assault, while others enter sexual relationships willingly, often due to promises of marriage, gifts, financial incentives, pressure from partners, or exploitation by older men. Most are unaware of the potential consequences or the need for contraception.

   Among middle- and upper-class adolescents, media sexualisation, exposure to Western cultural norms, and easy access to pornography contribute to the rising incidence of premarital sex. Curiosity, peer influence, and heightened libido are major contributing factors. In urban society, early puberty combined with delayed marriage creates a prolonged gap between biological readiness and legal or social consent, which may encourage premarital sexual activity.

2. **Early Marriage**

   In many Indian villages, early sexual activity occurs within the context of early marriage. Despite legal prohibitions, child marriage persists in certain regions as a social custom. While it places adolescent sexuality within socially sanctioned boundaries and may reduce premarital sexual activity, it carries serious consequences. Early marriage curtails education and vocational training, limiting a girl's socioeconomic development and confining her role to childbearing and caregiving. Even legitimate pregnancies at this age carry higher risks, as the body is not fully mature, leading to increased maternal and foetal complications. Psychologically, the adolescent is ill-equipped for parenthood.

Limited access to contraception, repeated pregnancies or abortions, and physically demanding labour further compromise her health. The result is the premature erosion of potential before it has fully emerged.

3. **Abstinence**

   Abstinence is declining globally. Adolescents who refrain from sexual intercourse may engage in masturbation and subsequently experience guilt due to persistent myths surrounding the practice. Such misconceptions cause unnecessary shame and distress. It is important for young people to understand that masturbation is neither harmful nor immoral. It is, in fact, the safest form of sexual expression.

Addressing Psychosexual Issues

Role of Parents

At the parental level, it is wise to be neither overly permissive nor excessively authoritarian; strike a balanced course. Assert authority clearly and consistently. Do not give in to persistent pleading; adolescents may exploit divisions between parents, making a united approach essential. Parents should remain aware of how their child spends their time, with whom, and where. Inviting their friends home, maintaining contact with their parents, and staying engaged allows for informed supervision. Warning signs, such as unexplained money, sudden lifestyle changes, or expensive gifts, should be taken seriously. Awareness of their daughter's menstrual patterns—especially her last menstrual period (LMP)—may also help identify concerns early. A missed period could mean a pregnancy, which—if discovered early—could be managed better.

Most importantly, ensure that she knows she has your support and can approach you with any problem, however serious. Education empowers her to achieve economic independence and reduces vulnerability to abusive relationships later in life. Parents have a duty to raise children into adults with sound physical, mental, emotional, social, and sexual health.

Adolescence is a time of identity formation—acknowledge her individuality, listen to her perspective, and respond reasonably. This fosters confidence and emotional resilience.

Role of Schools

Schools play a crucial role. Adolescents must have access to accurate, age-appropriate information. They should understand that high-risk sexual behaviour can result in STIs, chronic reproductive health conditions, and infertility. Educational institutions should also provide access to trained counsellors or social workers for confidential guidance. Zero tolerance towards sexual harassment must be enforced.

Role of Government

Government policy is central to adolescent reproductive health. This includes strict enforcement of minimum age-of-marriage laws, accessible counselling centres, non-judgemental healthcare services, and educational resources on safe sex and risk reduction. Clinics offering STI treatment, contraception, and safe abortion services must be easily accessible, staffed by professionals who treat adolescents with dignity and respect.

Role of Mass Media

Mass media has immense influence over young minds and therefore carries significant responsibility. In the absence of real-life role models, celebrities often fill the void. Film and television personalities must remain conscious of the values they project when showcasing their lifestyles.

To sum up, the adolescent, despite their defiant exterior, is often a confused and vulnerable individual in need of guidance and reassurance. Do not be deterred by unconventional hairstyles, sharp retorts or apparent indifference. Beneath the bravado lies a frightened child masking uncertainty with bravado. Set limits but remain present. Allow her to explore her identity cautiously while maintaining boundaries. Navigating the turbulent waters of adolescence is challenging, but it is our duty to ease the journey towards adulthood. The rewards—for both parent and child—are immeasurable.

12

When Sex Meets the Cycle

Let us begin with the taboos associated with sex during periods in different cultures and religions. Almost all have placed restrictions on sexual relations with a menstruating woman.

The Old Testament

According to the Old Testament, a menstruating woman is perceived as 'unclean' for seven days. Whoever touches her shall be unclean until evening, but 'if a man actually lies with her so that her menstrual impurity is on him, he shall be unclean seven days, and every bed on which he lies shall be unclean [Leviticus 15:24].'

In another biblical passage, it is stated that if a man has sexual relations with a woman during her menstrual period, both of them must be cut off from the community, for they have been exposed to the source of her blood flow. Men and women could regain purity by washing their clothes, bathing, or offering sacrifices [Leviticus 20:18].

These were essentially hygiene rules that were invested with religious authority. Their aim was to maintain the health of the community by decreasing the incidence of STIs, thereby increasing fertility and the likelihood of healthy offspring.

Christianity

The provisions of the Mosaic Law, as mentioned above, laid the basis for subsequent religions influenced by Judaism, namely Christianity and Islam. In the New Testament, Jesus did not oppose the supposed 'uncleanliness' of lepers and menstruating women; instead, he discouraged their exclusion from society by facilitating their access to God. According to him, 'The Sabbath was made for man, not man for the Sabbath [Mark 2:27–28].'

Early Christian church writings mention that 'neither lawful mixture, nor child-bearing, nor the menstrual purgation, nor nocturnal pollution can defile the nature of a man, or separate the Holy Spirit from him.'

According to Apostle Paul, these provisions are of no value for a man or woman renewed in Christ. They are not meant for the righteous but for lawless and rebellious persons, such as prostitutes. Here, 'prostitution' does not refer solely to sex work, but to any sexual act outside marriage or during menstruation—acts believed to be done for pleasure rather than for childbirth, which was considered the purpose of sex within marriage.

Islam

Islam also forbids men from having vaginal sexual intercourse with their wives during menstruation. In the Quran (2:222), Allah says: 'And they ask you about menstruation. Say, it is harm, so keep away from wives during menstruation. And when they have purified themselves, then come to them from where Allah has ordained for you.'

Hinduism

Traditionally, sexual intercourse during menstruation is forbidden due to the belief that menstrual blood is impure and may negatively affect the husband or potential offspring. Ayurveda advises against sex during menstruation, suggesting it may cause health issues such as pain, bloating, and infection.

Hindus and Jains usually do not allow a woman into the kitchen or temple during this period. Traditionally, she sleeps, cooks, and eats in a space away from the rest of the household, often a thatched hut. My Nepali helper once told me about a girl who was sent to such a dwelling during her period and died after being bitten by a snake!

However, whether viewed as pure or impure, this segregation does offer her rest from gruelling domestic chores, which the husband or other female members of the family take over—a luxury that an urban working woman in a nuclear family often cannot afford. However, the segregation of the menstruating woman is now seen as deeply sexist.

Tantric Practices

In contrast, Tantric traditions view menstruation as a sacred and powerful time, associating it with the divine feminine and the creative force of nature. Sexual activity during menstruation is included as part of ritualistic spiritual practice.

Modern Medical Approach

Modern medicine considers sex during menstruation normal and not a perversion. Benefits include pain relief, as orgasm can ease menstrual cramps, and enhanced pleasure due to increased blood flow and heightened sensitivity. Many couples report increased intimacy after this experience. Commonly preferred positions for sex during periods include spooning, missionary, cowgirl, and reverse cowgirl.

Harmful effects may include STIs if intercourse is performed without a condom during or shortly after menstruation, as blood provides a favourable medium for microorganisms to grow. The loss of the protective cervical mucus plug, a slightly dilated cervical opening, and the alkaline pH of the vagina are other contributory factors. There is an increased risk of infections such as chlamydia, a preventable cause of pelvic inflammatory disease (PID) that can silently but permanently damage and block the fallopian tubes, leading to infertility. Gonorrhoea can have a similar effect on the female genital tract, but symptoms such as burning while passing urine and greenish-yellow vaginal discharge often prompt earlier treatment.

Sex during periods may lead to increased menstrual flow due to congestion of uterine vessels, or periods may stop a day or two earlier, as the uterine contractions induced by orgasm help expel menstrual blood sooner.

Although the chances of pregnancy after unprotected sex during menstruation are low, it is not unheard of. Sperm can survive within a woman's body for several days, and women with a short menstrual cycle of around 21 days may ovulate soon after their periods, resulting in unintended conception.

There is also a remote possibility of endometriosis—a disorder characterised by the presence of endometrial tissue outside the uterine cavity. Rhythmic contractions of the uterus during orgasm may push menstrual blood, along with endometrial tissue, into the fallopian tubes, from where it can enter the pelvic cavity and implant on the ovaries or peritoneum, leading to pelvic pain and infertility.

Many men may be reluctant to engage in vaginal intercourse during periods due to the presence of blood, which can be messy, and the associated odour. Premenstrual syndrome (PMS), cramps, anxiety, low mood, and migraines may also dampen desire in both partners. However, if sex during menstruation is something a couple enjoys, it is important to use barrier methods such as condoms to protect against STIs and unintended pregnancy.

Taboos associated with menstruation should not make a woman feel guilty or ashamed; she is in no way unclean. A healthy attitude and respect towards her body must be cultivated. Sex during menstruation is not a perversion, but responsible behaviour is encouraged. As Apostle Paul stated: 'Everything is permissible for me, but not everything is beneficial.'

13

Intimacy during Pregnancy

Shivani was a credit to Indian femininity. Tall and slim, with a wheatish complexion, an oval face, and a ready smile, she was the traditional Indian *bahu*. A thick black plait snaked down her back, visible through the translucent organza of the sari *pallu* that covered her head. It had been a fairy-tale wedding. They had gone to see the girl in Moradabad and had returned with the bride—just like that. She was merely nineteen years old and had become pregnant soon after marriage, hence the visit to the gynaecologist.

I found the girl immensely likeable. I could well understand how the magnetic appeal of her big black eyes had made the boy and his family behave as romantically as they did. During the antenatal visits that followed, I got to know her better. When she came with her *jethani* (husband's elder brother's wife), Rajni, an old patient of mine, Shivani was the demure *bahu* with downcast eyes. On the days she came with her husband, she was bubbly, playful, and talkative. Love shone from his eyes as he indulged her.

One day, Rajni came alone to discuss a rather embarrassing issue regarding Shivani. According to her, the girl was excessively interested in sex. Even in her delicate condition, she wanted intercourse every day, much to her brother-in-law's discomfort. He worried that something might happen to the baby and refused to oblige, which led to quarrels in bed.

She concluded her tirade with, '*Naya, naya khoon muh laga hai* (she has newly tasted blood).'

I laughed and asked, 'Did your *devar* [husband's younger brother] complain to you?'

'No! He is very respectful and does not even look me in the eye. He told my husband, who in turn asked me to discuss the matter with you.'

So, the next time she came for an antenatal visit, I asked Shivani to reduce her nocturnal activities, though she needn't stop them altogether. In all probability, the baby would not come to harm, but as in all other aspects of life, moderation was key.

Then disaster struck. Shivani went into premature labour. All our efforts to stop the labour pains were in vain. She delivered a tiny baby girl who was shifted to a tertiary care unit. After two months in the nursery and a series of serious complications, the baby succumbed to necrotising enterocolitis, leaving the family poorer by a couple of lakhs. Shivani did not shed a tear. As expected, her in-laws blamed her for this catastrophe.

Sex during pregnancy was, until recently, a taboo subject due to our tendency to dissociate sex from motherhood. From a medical point of view, sexual intercourse and orgasm during a normal pregnancy do not harm the foetus. The couple can continue to have intercourse right up to the onset of labour. Traditionally, women are told to avoid sex during the first three months and in the later months, and most couples abide by this unwritten rule. This is particularly hard on newlyweds and newly pregnant couples still in their honeymoon period.

I remember the case of a woman with threatened abortion[15]. As she had vaginal spotting, I forbade intercourse and prescribed the requisite treatment. Her husband whispered something in her ear and walked out.

'He wants to know if we could do it from behind,' asked the embarrassed wife.

'Behind or front, the opening is the same.'

'No, he means the opening at the back,' she clarified.

My nurse ran out, trying to stifle her laughter with her hand over her mouth. Anal intercourse, too, was inadvisable, as orgasm could lead to uterine contractions that might expel the pregnancy.

Just because sex is permitted during pregnancy does not mean that the woman wants it. Desire for sex during pregnancy varies from person to person. In some women, like Shivani, it increases, while others are averse to the idea of intercourse. The husband should not feel rejected, for it is not about him but about her hormones, which dictate her libido. Fearing harm to the pregnancy or burdened with the responsibilities of impending fatherhood, some husbands avoid sex. The wife should not feel that, because she has become ungainly, he no longer desires her. Everyone reacts differently to a given situation, and one should not take it personally. Communication is key; be open with each other and express your feelings freely. Moreover, there is nothing to stop the husband from being kind and caring. Intimate talks, tender kisses, and cuddles strengthen the marital bond, and the negligible sex life will cease to matter.

In the first trimester, the pregnant woman may experience morning sickness, fatigue, frequent urination, and breast tenderness, which makes her lose interest in sex. The interest may return—perhaps with gusto—during the middle three months, when these symptoms subside and the woman is more than ready to make up for lost time. Freedom from contraceptive concerns, combined with a renewed sense of closeness with her partner, makes sex more fulfilling.

As the abdomen enlarges in the third trimester, intercourse should be done in positions that put less pressure on it, such as spooning or facing each other when the baby bump is small. In later months, the man could enter her from behind while lying down or with the woman on all fours. The woman could opt for the woman-on-top position, as she can control the depth of penetration. Some women experience a diminished desire for sex in the last months as they are preoccupied with preparations for the new arrival.

Sex, masturbation, and even nipple stimulation must be avoided if there is a history of miscarriages or premature labour, if the woman is carrying twins, if there is pain in the lower abdomen, vaginal bleeding, or leakage of fluid. The bleeding could be due to threatened abortion in early pregnancy, placental abruption (blood clot between the placenta and uterus), and placenta praevia—when the placenta occupies the lower part of the uterus (the last two are complications of later pregnancy). In all these cases, sex is a definite no. In cases of cervical incompetence, a weak cervix unable to hold the growing foetus—which can lead to late miscarriage—sex is prohibited.

On the other hand, if the due date has been crossed and there is no sign of labour, one can have sex and/or stimulate the nipples to induce labour.

Two types of sexual behaviour are unsafe in any pregnancy at any time. These are sex with an unknown or multiple partners, as there is a very real risk of STIs that can harm the pregnancy. In fact, it is advisable to have sex with a condom even if both partners are HIV positive, to reduce viral load. Blowing air into the vagina should be avoided, as this could lead to air embolism, a condition that could be fatal.

Sex usually does not harm the baby, for it is contained within the bag of waters; moreover, the mouth of the uterus is a tightly closed tube, about 4 cm long, sealed with a thick mucus plug. The penis does not come in contact with the baby; however, as mentioned earlier, orgasmic uterine contractions may cause issues. If there is bleeding, pain, or discharge from the vagina after sex, inform your doctor immediately.

14

Rediscovering Intimacy after Childbirth

Who on earth coined the phrase 'slept like a baby'? Try telling that to a new mother, and she will throw a pillow at your face, fumed Radhika.

The baby barely slept for an hour or two, and by the time she finished a bath and organised her things, he was yelling his lungs out for his next feed. Ever since his birth, life had been a whirl of smelly diapers, red bottoms, shrill cries, and an ever-hungry mouth that led to painfully sore nipples. As for the haggard apparition that stared back at her in the mirror, Radhika was horror-struck.

This woman, in a crumpled nightie two sizes too big for her, with dishevelled hair, a weary face, and dark circles under her sleep-deprived eyes, couldn't be me! thought Radhika, ready to pull her hair out in frustration. Where were those sweet babies who slept peacefully in cribs (this one clung to her like a little monkey), with svelte, perfectly coiffured mothers cooing ecstatically over them, as seen in baby product ads that beguile would-be mothers? Viciously, she ripped open the buttons of her nightie to reveal swollen, blue-veined breasts and a sagging, wrinkled, striae-streaked belly, laying bare the stark contrast between fantasy and the reality of a new mother, and dissolved into a spell of crying.

Perhaps she would not have felt so low if she had help; even a mother-in-law was welcome during these trying times. To think that, only a short while ago, she felt lucky to live in a nuclear family without interfering in-laws—both were dead. The japa caregiver who was to come from Kolkata to help her tide over the forty-day lying-in period ditched her at the last moment, and her part-time help was, well, part-time.

At her six-week postnatal visit, the gynaecologist examined her and told her that everything was fine.

'As for your periods,' she continued, 'they may start right away or could be delayed for as long as a year, especially if you are breastfeeding your baby. However, you can resume sexual activity now, but remember, pregnancy can occur before your cycles resume. So, this is as good a time as any to talk about contraception.'

'Thanks, but no thanks. You have already provided us with a 24/7 contraceptive.'

'Which one?' asked the doctor, perplexed, for she had done no such thing.

'This live, wailing, and kicking one,' said Radhika, holding out her baby. 'Whatever little time His Highness deigns to give me, I would rather sleep.'

'I understand,' said the doctor after they had stopped laughing, 'but years of practice have shown me that those who do not opt for contraception now come back within a year for an abortion and contraceptive advice.'

'I'll be leaving for my parents' place this weekend and will stay there for two months. I'll get back to you when I return.'

'The least you can do is keep condoms handy, for by the time your husband comes to pick you up, you'll be ready for sex after months of abstinence and are likely to conceive. We will talk about more effective contraceptives after your return.'

Life at her mother's place was bliss. Her parents took turns looking after the baby, fed him expressed breast milk, and let her sleep away her exhaustion. This allowed her mind and body (including her nipples) to heal. Rested and refreshed, she actually began to feel kindly towards the baby she had resented all along. Mother–child bonding was restored, never to be broken again, at least from her side, in her lifetime. The baby, too, developed a proper sleep–food cycle, and life became that much easier. Radhika was overwhelmed with gratitude for her mother, not only for taking care of her baby but because she realised what her mother had gone through for her—a realisation that sons will never have.

Days passed, but strange are the ways of nature. No matter how comfortable a girl is at her mother's place, a time comes when she wants to go back home, to the home she has made with her husband. This did not upset her parents, for that was how it was supposed to be. The day her husband was coming to pick her up, Radhika waited for him all spruced up, with a *gajra* in her hair, a smile on her lips, and a content baby asleep in her arms. Neither of them could wait for night to fall. Her understanding parents took their grandson to sleep with them, ostensibly to spend as much time as they could with him before he left, though partly it was to allow the sex-deprived couple a night of bliss.

Thanks to them, the time was well utilised, though with a few glitches. Her husband felt as if he were cohabiting with a new Radhika. Though she had been diligently performing Kegel exercises to get her vaginal muscles back in shape, she did need extra lubrication to overcome the discomfort of penetration, for she had been warned that a certain amount of postpartum dryness was to be expected due to hormonal changes.

⚤

Now for a bit of the didactic. The genital tract remains tender for several weeks after childbirth and needs time to recover. Though episiotomy stitches heal within 10–14 days, they are still too raw to allow vaginal penetration. Traditionally, sex is forbidden for forty days, till the body, especially the genitalia, returns to normal. One wonders how on earth our ancestors knew. Doctors tend to agree with the four-to-six-week period of abstinence, for it allows complete healing and the return of the genital organs to their pre-pregnant state. If one does have sex before this time, there are increased chances of bleeding and infection, which could delay healing.

Due to hormonal changes, a woman may either feel intense love for her partner and an increased libido—especially if there have been months of abstinence during pregnancy—or lose interest in sex after delivery. This could be due to fatigue, sleep deprivation, anxiety over baby care, or hormonal shifts. Her partner should not feel rejected; it is not about him. I would advise the husband not to rush her. Be patient, caring, and intimate in other ways. Cuddle, cosy up, and help with the baby so she can catch up on her sleep.

However, if a lack of interest persists, or if she experiences mood swings, loss of appetite, or a general disinterest in the baby and life, this could indicate postpartum depression, which needs to be taken seriously. A psychiatric consultation is warranted.

It is also important to remember that sex after childbirth is never going to be exactly as it was before. Pregnancy, labour, and vaginal delivery can stretch or injure the pelvic floor muscles, making the vagina feel lax; this can be improved with Kegel exercises.

Even after a prolonged period of abstinence, sex may feel different, and somewhat uncomfortable at first—even after a caesarean section. This is particularly true if the woman is breastfeeding, her periods have not resumed, or she is using hormonal contraception. A decrease in oestrogen levels can lead to vaginal dryness and painful intercourse. The husband should be gentle, considerate, and begin with nonsexual foreplay, such as a massage, which can feel good after all the exertion of labour and make her more receptive. Spend ample time on foreplay and use plenty of lubricant to make penetration smooth. If there is pain or discomfort, especially where stitches are present, her body is not yet ready, and sexual activity should be delayed. In such situations, couples can explore mutual masturbation or oral sex. Every woman and every couple is different, and open communication usually resolves most issues. If problems persist, medical advice should be sought.

Additionally, special care is needed after a caesarean. Physical recovery of the internal genitalia is similar for both vaginal and caesarean deliveries, so intercourse should be delayed for six weeks in both cases. Kegel exercises are not just for the vagina but for the entire pelvic floor, which stretches during pregnancy, regardless of delivery type. These exercises should therefore be done post-caesarean as well.

Vaginal dryness can occur after a caesarean, and liberal use of lubricant may be necessary. The abdominal incision may still be tender, so care should be taken to avoid pressure on it during sex. Comfortable sexual positions after a caesarean include side by side facing each other, spooning with rear entry, or woman on top—allowing control over penetration depth and avoiding contact with the abdomen. Positions that put pressure on the caesarean scar should be avoided until fully healed. Doggy style may strain core muscles and the pelvic area.

Whatever the mode of delivery, if the initial sexual experience is unpleasant, the memory of pain can create fear. If the husband forces intercourse, resentment can develop, leading to a vicious cycle.

Some women may feel insecure, thinking their husbands no longer find them attractive due to changes in their body—flabby muscles, a crumpled abdomen, or vaginal laxity. One should not be ashamed of a body that has accomplished something extraordinary: Nurturing and delivering a new life is nothing short of a miracle, and a thoughtful partner should appreciate it. That said, for the sake of self-esteem and health, postnatal exercises, yoga, and diet modifications can help regain pre-pregnancy fitness.

Breastfeeding does not spoil breast shape. Nursing generously benefits the baby, helps the uterus return to its original size (thanks to oxytocin, which also promotes sexual arousal), and can accelerate weight loss, as body fat is transferred to the baby through milk. Mothers who breastfeed also have a lower risk of breast cancer.

For women with significant vaginal laxity, surgical options exist to reduce the size of the vaginal orifice, typically performed 3–6 months after delivery and ideally after completing the family. However, for most women, Kegel exercises suffice. These involve contracting and relaxing the vaginal muscles as if stopping urination midstream. They improve tone and elasticity, restoring the vagina to near pre-delivery condition. Devices such as the Kegella chair are available in some hospitals to aid these exercises.

Nonsurgical methods, discussed in aesthetic gynaecology, can also help restore vaginal size and shape and address issues like urinary leakage that some women experience after childbirth.

Contraception

During your postnatal visit, your doctor will also discuss contraception—and rightly so. The last thing a newly delivered woman wants is another pregnancy, though constant baby care, sleep deprivation, and fatigue are not conducive to sexual activity. Some nursing mothers experience lactational amenorrhea (absence of periods while breastfeeding), which suppresses ovulation and acts as a natural contraceptive of sorts. However, one cannot rely on it entirely because ovulation can occur before menstruation resumes.

To allow the mother to recover fully from childbirth and ensure adequate care for the newborn, the ideal interval between two pregnancies is three years. This means that some form of contraception is necessary. Fortunately, there are various options to choose from.

Condoms

This is the simplest contraceptive method, acting as a mechanical barrier. Condoms are safe, reversible, and have minimal side effects (such as latex allergy). However, they have a higher failure rate due to breakage or leakage, which is a concern in the postnatal period. Some couples feel that condoms interfere with enjoyment, either because the act is interrupted to put them on or because skin-to-skin contact is reduced—aptly described by a patient as 'like eating a toffee with the wrapper on'. Condoms also protect against STIs. Additionally, female condoms are available as well.

Oral Contraceptive Pills (OCPs)

Except in certain medical conditions, most women can use OCPs. When taken regularly as prescribed, the chances of pregnancy are negligible. These pills contain low-dose oestrogen and progesterone, which prevent ovulation. Irregular intake can cause intermittent spotting or even pregnancy.

OCPs are especially beneficial for women with menstrual irregularities, painful periods, or PMS, as these symptoms are often alleviated. Side effects are generally minimal but may include bloating, weight gain, headaches, or nausea. OCPs are contraindicated in women with a history of jaundice, liver disease, blood clots, or other specific conditions, which a specialist will review before prescribing.

After delivery, progesterone-only pills are recommended, as oestrogens can reduce milk production and increase the risk of blood clots during the postnatal hypercoagulable state. Progesterone-only injections may be given every three months but can cause menstrual irregularities, including the cessation of periods.

Many are aware of emergency contraceptive pills, which prevent pregnancy if taken within 72 hours of unprotected intercourse. The success rate is about 85 per cent, but they can cause menstrual irregularities. They should not be relied upon as a regular contraceptive method.

Intrauterine Contraceptive Devices (IUCDs)

An IUCD is a small, copper-containing device inserted into the uterus. The copper alters the uterine environment, preventing implantation of a fertilised egg. IUCDs must be inserted by a healthcare provider and they offer protection for 3–10 years, depending on the type. They are ideal for spacing pregnancies. Hormone-containing IUCDs are available for women with menstrual irregularities.

Side effects may include pain, prolonged or heavy periods, and pre- or post-menstrual spotting during the first few cycles, as the uterus adjusts to the device. Rare complications include expulsion, ectopic pregnancy, or migration into the abdominal cavity. Despite these risks, IUCDs remain an excellent contraceptive option.

Permanent Methods

Permanent contraception may be chosen when childbearing is complete. Men can undergo vasectomy, while women may have their fallopian tubes ligated. Vasectomy is simpler to perform, but some men resist, mistakenly equating fertility with potency.

Laparoscopic female sterilisation involves a small abdominal incision and is generally more acceptable to women, who bear the physical burden of repeated pregnancies and childbirth. Sterilisation can also be performed via an open method after delivery or caesarean or following medical termination of pregnancy.

Though called permanent, these methods can fail occasionally. On the other hand, it is not easy to reverse a permanent form of contraception. Recanalisation of the Fallopian tubes is a major plastic surgery that is not always successful; though, some women may desire it for reasons such as loss of a child or remarriage.

As we have seen, there is a wide range of contraceptive options, and the choice depends on individual preference and medical considerations. Medicine is not mathematics, and no method is 100 per cent effective. Side effects are usually mild and manageable, and negligible compared to the stress of an unwanted pregnancy or the consequences of abortion. Couples should discuss the pros and cons of each option with a specialist. Once comfortable with a chosen method, there is no reason why they cannot enjoy an active, healthy, and stress-free sex life.

15

Menopause and Sexual Well-Being

It takes all kinds to make up this world. This holds true for the desire for sex, or the lack of it, in postmenopausal women. Some look forward to an unencumbered love life; others feel ashamed of having such desires at 'this age' and try to repress them, while yet others manage very well without sex. If, due to cultural conditioning, religious beliefs, psychosomatic concerns, or marital issues, some women would like to abstain from sex, it is entirely their prerogative. Decreased libido, vaginal dryness leading to pain during intercourse, illnesses such as diabetes and hypertension, orthopaedic problems, medications, or an ageing or unwell partner with erectile dysfunction also contribute to a state of celibacy during this period.

A boy once questioned his grandfather about whether he still had intimate relations with his grandmother.

'Yes,' said the old man, with a twinkle in his eye.

'Wow!' exclaimed the boy, impressed. 'Missionary style, I presume . . .' for that was all he thought older people were capable of.

'No, I prefer oral sex.'

'What?'

'Well, before going to bed, I tell her, "I fu*k you", and she says the same to me, and we go off to sleep in each other's arms.'

This salacious bit of humour highlights the fact that if both partners are comfortable without sex at this phase of their lives, it is perfectly fine. With gestures such as holding hands, kissing, and cuddling, a loving relationship is maintained.

By and large, sexuality exists well beyond menopause. In fact, some couples seem to enjoy it more during this period than in their heyday. This is because there is no fear of pregnancy, child-rearing is a thing of the past, and the mad rush of youth is over. Retired, both child-wise and job-wise, the couple finally has the house to themselves and all the time in the world to do what they want. However, mind-blowing orgasms and all-night marathons are neither a possibility nor on their list of priorities. Even if sex is restricted to infrequent, tentative efforts or mutual masturbation, the sense of well-being and closeness remains the same.

A woman's sexual response to her partner, however, depends on the quality of her sex life before menopause. If it was not satisfying earlier, the situation is unlikely to improve now. There are postmenopausal women who retain a healthy interest in sex but are unable to find an outlet, either because they are single or their partner is unable to satisfy them. In such cases, there should be no guilt in taking matters into one's own hands, both literally and figuratively, for there is nothing shameful or sinful about self-gratification.

The sexual response after menopause may take the following forms:

- Normal desire in both partners and satisfactory sex, which can continue as before
- Normal desire but painful intercourse
- Decreased or absent libido
- Increased libido

Pain during Intercourse

Soreness, pain, itching, and cuts during intercourse are the most common reasons women abstain from sex at this age. This occurs because decreased levels of female sex hormones lead to reduced blood supply to the genitals, causing the vagina to lose its moisture and elasticity and become thin and dry. Friction during intercourse can lead to severe pain, which puts a woman off sex completely.

There is no need to lose heart or desire on this account, as remedies are available. If the soreness is mild, the application of water-based lubricants such as KY Jelly before intercourse can make life more enjoyable. Oil-based lubricants such as petroleum jelly should be avoided, as they provide a medium for bacterial growth and also weaken latex condoms.

'Condoms after menopause?' one might ask, amazed. However, postmenopausal women need contraception for at least two years after the cessation of periods, as erratic ovulation can still occur, and she could end up becoming a mother instead of a grandmother. Moreover, condoms provide protection against STIs that may be acquired from a new or unfaithful partner. In fact, one must be wary of new or multiple sexual partners at this age, as the thin, dry vaginal mucosa is easily bruised, increasing the risk of infection.

If lubricants do not help, a gynaecologist may prescribe oestrogen cream for local application to help the vagina regain some of its moisture and elasticity, thereby improving sexual comfort. It also reduces burning and itching and helps prevent infections.

Poor Libido

Here, too, declining oestrogen levels are often the culprit. Despite the best efforts of her partner, a woman may not be as easily aroused by foreplay as before, which can make him feel inadequate. He may feel hurt by her lack of interest, or what he perceives as a lack of interest, which can lead to emotional distance and a disturbed relationship. He should understand that it is not always about him. If pain and dryness are the underlying issues, oestrogen creams, as already mentioned, can help. Other contributing factors include poor bladder control, sleep disturbances, depression or anxiety, systemic illnesses, and medications taken for other conditions. If the couple is distressed by her lack of sexual desire, menopausal hormone therapy (MHT) may be considered under strict medical supervision. Testosterone patches are also being explored to improve sexual health and desire.

Increased Libido

'Increased libido at this age?' one might ask incredulously. Yet it is possible. Women have small amounts of testosterone in their bodies, which plays a role in libido. After menopause, declining female hormone levels allow circulating testosterone to have a greater effect, sometimes increasing sex drive. It is also responsible for postmenopausal hirsutism, which explains why some older women develop coarse hair on the chin or upper lip.

An increased interest in sex may also stem from the absence of fear of pregnancy, reduced need for contraception, relief from the fatigue of child-rearing, and easing of job-related stress after retirement. Most importantly, the couple has time, privacy, and constant access to one another. This can be liberating for a postmenopausal woman. What advice can one give her other than to enjoy it, provided her partner is up to the 'new' her?

This quote sums up the sexuality of middle-aged women beautifully:

> Once you get past a wrinkle or two, an older woman is far sexier than her younger counterpart. Her libido is stronger, her fear of pregnancy gone. Her experience of lovemaking is honed and reciprocal, and she knows how to please a man in ways her daughter could never dream of. (Young men, you have something to look forward to.)
>
> **—Andy Rooney**

16

Sex and Health Conditions

There are several couples out there whose sex life is disturbed due to an illness in one partner. Many of them resign themselves to a life without sex or seek pleasure elsewhere. These need not necessarily be the only options available to them. It is possible to enjoy a reasonably good sex life after debilitating illnesses like cancer and paralysis. Let's take them up one by one.

Sex after Cancer

During the initial stages, when fear and numbness overwhelm, sex is farthest from the mind of a person with cancer. Decreased sexual function is also a side effect of certain cancers, such as uterine, cervical, ovarian, and breast cancer. As time passes and patients learn to live with their illness, many seek advice about sex and intimacy. The sense of well-being and release that sex offers is not something one wishes to forgo. Moreover, intimacy reiterates the fact that they are as desirable and loved as before. However, most are too embarrassed to seek advice on such a delicate matter.

Discussing intimate issues with female healthcare providers is often easier than opening up to male doctors; therefore, a compassionate woman doctor should initiate the conversation herself. Although a gynaecologist or oncologist may not be an expert on sexual health, she can explain the side effects of procedures such as the removal of the ovaries or pelvic irradiation, which can be immediate and profound. As a woman is abruptly thrust into a postmenopausal state, she should be prepared for menopausal symptoms that, among other effects, lead to decreased libido, vaginal thinning, and dryness resulting in painful penetration (dyspareunia), all of which may adversely affect her sex life. After treatment is completed, she can be referred to specialists such as sex therapists or couples' counsellors.

There are also women who are aghast at their partner's desire for sex while they are going through such a critical period in their lives. Social, cultural, religious, and interpersonal factors come into play. Decreased interest in sex may persist long after cancer treatment is over and can itself be a side effect of cancer management. Radiation therapy may lead to narrowing of the vagina. Pre-existing conditions such as diabetes also contribute to reduced sexual desire, as does overall fitness. Low libido is a frequent complaint across all cancer types, particularly among breast cancer patients on certain medications and is not limited to cancers involving the ovaries.

Then there are women who are BRCA 1 and BRCA 2 positive and therefore at high risk of developing breast and ovarian cancer. Many undergo prophylactic removal of the fallopian tubes and ovaries, leading to severe and abrupt menopausal symptoms. Based on the Female Sexual Function Index (FSFI), which assesses desire, arousal, lubrication, orgasm, satisfaction, and pain, women who had their ovaries removed fared poorly across several domains.[16]

Patients with dyspareunia may benefit from lubricants or vaginal oestrogen creams, depending on the severity of burning, itching, irritation, tissue fragility, and pain during intercourse. Those with deep dyspareunia can use penile bumpers to limit the depth of penetration. Keeping the legs straight, instead of raising them, also decreases the depth of penile penetration. Vaginal dilators may be used to prevent stenosis following radiation therapy. Researchers are also exploring ways to shield the clitoris from radiation exposure in order to preserve sexual function.

Nowadays, before irradiation for cancers of the pelvic region, like the uterus and the rectum, the ovaries are transposed and fixed surgically at a point above the pelvis, in the abdomen, so that they are spared the side effect of radiation.

Sexual Challenges in Childhood Cancer Survivors (CCS)

With improved treatment modalities, more than 80 to 85 per cent of children diagnosed with cancer now survive into adulthood. Many experience long-term physical and psychological issues; sexual dysfunction is a common and significant late effect, as both cancer and its treatment interfere with normal physiological, psychological, and sexual development. This often leads to difficulties in forming or sustaining romantic relationships. Some survivors never experience sexual attraction or feel sexually desirable. Poorer sexual health outcomes are more common among female survivors and vary depending on the type of cancer, the treatment received, and the age at diagnosis. Those diagnosed in early childhood generally fare better than those diagnosed during adolescence.

Sex after a Heart Attack or Stenting

One of the foremost questions in the mind of a person who has survived a heart attack or undergone stenting for blocked coronary arteries is, 'When can I have sex?'

Although sex and intimacy are vital to emotional well-being, many people hesitate to ask, fearing that the doctor may judge them for thinking about sex after narrowly escaping death. Reassurance is warranted: Doctors are generally open to answering such questions, and the more empathetic ones often initiate the conversation themselves.

It is generally safe to resume sexual activity after a heart attack, bypass surgery, or stenting, once recovery is underway. The timing depends on the severity of the heart attack, the treatment received, coexisting illnesses, overall health, and libido. Men and women who have had a mild heart attack or uncomplicated stenting can usually resume sexual activity after a couple of weeks. In fact, sex may have positive effects on heart health by reducing stress and promoting a sense of well-being. Resuming sexual activity within the first few months after a heart attack may even improve long-term survival.

However, it is advisable to ease back gradually, starting with less strenuous positions.

Those who have had a severe heart attack or heart surgery will require more time to recover, typically six to eight weeks. If symptoms such as chest pain, shortness of breath, or irregular heartbeat occur during or after sexual activity, one should stop and seek medical advice. Masturbation or oral stimulation can place similar demands on the heart and should also be avoided until deemed safe. In the interim, holding hands, kissing, cuddling, and romantic outings help the affected partner feel wanted and loved, fostering emotional well-being. If a person can perform moderate physical activity, such as climbing two flights of stairs without symptoms, they are generally fit enough for sex. A doctor may also recommend a stress test to assess fitness levels.

When resuming sexual activity, ensure a relaxed, interruption-free environment. Slow, prolonged foreplay allows heart rate and blood pressure to rise gradually. Choose positions that require less exertion, such as the missionary or seated position. After open-heart surgery, avoid pressure on the chest. Sexual activity should also be avoided after alcohol consumption, heavy meals, within two to three hours of eating, and in extreme temperatures.

If it is the partner who has had the heart attack, roles may reverse, and erectile dysfunction may occur due to medications or anxiety. Heart disease itself can reduce blood flow to the genitals, leading to arousal and orgasmic difficulties. Self-medication to improve sexual performance is unsafe and should be avoided.

Paralysis and Sex

I love plants, which led me to befriend a botanist in my neighbourhood who lived with his paralysed wife. His terrace garden was lush and vibrant, in stark contrast to the dark, sombre atmosphere of his bedroom. I sat beside his wife. Her cropped grey hair, ivory skin, beautiful brown eyes, asymmetrical face, and the paralysed right side of her body intrigued me. She had been in this state for the past three years. Although devastatingly disabling, the condition was not always fatal; a friend's father had survived for twenty years.

I held her hand and spoke to her as I would to anyone else, though she could only stare back with her limpid eyes. After a while, she made a guttural sound, which her husband interpreted as a need to urinate. In front of me, he asked her caregiver to assist her. What I had thought was merely a wheelchair turned out to be a dual-purpose device. When the seat was removed, a commode was revealed. Right there, she relieved herself. The sound and smell were overwhelming. It took all my willpower not to reveal my revulsion, and I forced myself to finish my tea in that malodorous room.

Then, unexpectedly, her husband said something that jolted me.

'She has become oversexed, and I am unable to satisfy her.'

'What?' I spluttered.

Paralysis, and especially the sexual lives of people living with it, was not something I had ever given much thought to. I had perhaps assumed that loss of sensation meant an end to sexual desire.

As I tried to process this, he implored, 'Is there something you can do?'

I looked at the woman and found her staring at her husband, her eyes blazing.

'What are you so angry about? She is a doctor, and I am seeking her advice,' he told her.

What made him think a gynaecologist would have an answer to this question, I do not know.

'I am not the right person to answer this. Why don't you consult her neurologist?' I said, trying to keep the shock out of my voice. Then, prompted by curiosity, I asked, 'How do you know she wants intimacy?'

'She loosens the drawstrings of her salwar and pulls it down with her good hand. I am seventy; my libido is not what it used to be. How much Viagra can I take to please her? I heard it is bad for the heart.'

'Please ask her neurologist,' I repeated gently. He was clearly in a terrible predicament. As for the woman, she may have been unable to control her impulses, and I felt deeply sorry for her.

There is life after paralysis, often a long one, but how many of us pause to consider sexuality after paralysis? Back home, I immersed myself in medical journals in search of answers.

Post-stroke sexuality remains a taboo subject, and as a result, sexual rehabilitation in paralysed patients has been poorly studied. Sexual recovery after stroke needs to be addressed and integrated into rehabilitation programmes, although many healthcare professionals remain ill-informed on the subject. Stroke can affect female sexual functioning in various ways, depending on the location of the lesion, pre-existing comorbidities, and medications. Sexual difficulties present before the stroke often worsen afterwards.

Stroke frequently results in female sexual dysfunction. Many women experience absent or diminished genital sensation, affecting sexual pleasure, while others retain sensation but have difficulty achieving orgasm. Although hyposexuality is more common, some patients present with hypersexuality. Lesions in brain regions involved in sexual behaviour, such as the temporal or frontal lobes, can disrupt impulse control, leading to disinhibition and inappropriate sexual behaviour. Bipolar disorder may also cause hypersexuality, resulting in relationship difficulties. Identifying underlying causes, adopting appropriate management strategies, and setting boundaries are essential.

With increasing life expectancy and the rise in lifestyle-related diseases, it is sobering to realise that more people will live for years with paralysis. Disruptions in conjugal life and relationship challenges are inevitable, and sexual adjustments can strain even the strongest marriages. Understanding and compassionate healthcare professionals are the need of the hour.

Part III

Ancient Treatises on Sex

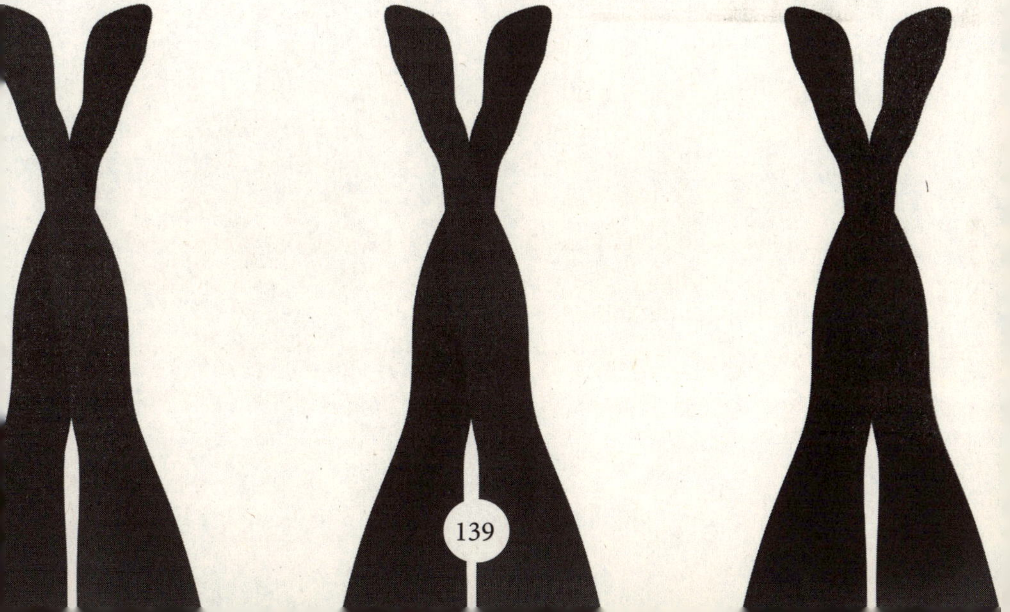

17

Kama Sutra: The Art of Love

A sage, Vatsyayana, wrote the *Kama Sutra* two thousand years ago. Yes, a *sage* crafted this cult classic. It is not only about sixty-four coital positions (some of which would challenge a contortionist) but also about the art of making love—an art that begins long before coitus, even before one touches the woman or speaks with her. Vatsyayana abstained from intercourse for the year it took him to write the *Kama Sutra*.

When Parvati despaired of gaining the attention of the meditating ascetic Shiva, Kama, the god of erotic love, tried to intervene on her behalf—and was burnt to ashes. No longer distracted by lust, Shiva told Parvati to ask for a boon. Promptly, she asked for the resurrection of Kama, for without him, 'there can be between man and woman no emotion like ten million suns.' Shiva granted her wish, restoring desire to the cosmos, and consummated his union with Parvati as part of the divine order.

According to Vatsyayana, the four tenets of the Hindu religion are: *Dharma* (right conduct), *Artha* (the acquisition of wealth), *Kama* (the pursuit of desire), and—if these three are pursued in balance—*Moksha* (salvation), the fourth and final goal, will automatically follow.

Critics of his work argued that sex was a basic instinct, shared even by animals, and questioned the need for such an elaborate manual. Vatsyayana countered that animals engage in sex solely for procreation, and only when the female is in heat, whereas humans copulate at all times; therefore, people need to understand how to obtain maximum pleasure from their bodies. By stating that desire is desirable, Vatsyayana absolved it of shame and guilt.

Once this issue was resolved, the sage set out to ensure that men became accomplished lovers. In an age when women were often treated as mere sexual objects or procreators, Vatsyayana proclaimed that female desire was no less than a man's, and it was his duty to lead her to the heights of sexual fulfilment. Mind-boggling as it may seem, he also understood the fundamental difference between male and female arousal: Men are quickly aroused and easily satisfied, whereas women require investment of time, effort, and expertise—but once aroused, she could leave the man 'limp at the post'.

The keyword here is 'aroused'. By mastering the art of female arousal, a man will not only enhance his own enjoyment but also gain her love and respect for life. A satisfying sexual encounter guarantees the next. One who uses a woman merely for personal gratification is the worst kind of lover. Sadly, most men, especially in our rushed modern times, lack the inclination, knowledge, and patience for prolonged foreplay. The unsatisfied woman may seek fulfilment elsewhere. Conversely, if a woman wishes her man to remain faithful, she should keep him satisfied, yet panting for more.

Preparations for a mutually satisfying sexual experience begin long before the act itself. A pleasing appearance (not necessarily a handsome face or bulging biceps), a sense of style, a subtle perfume, and impeccable manners incline a woman towards a man. A look, a compliment, or an intelligent conversation to keep her engaged is essential. A sense of humour and the gift of repartee are major plus points, as are music, dance, poetry, and the ability to give a good massage. It is unreasonable to expect every man to be this accomplished, but anyone can be presentable, smell pleasant, show courtesy, and take a genuine interest in her life. This reassures a woman that he values her as a person, not merely as a sexual object—a point of great importance to her.

Women, too, should pay attention to hygiene, dress, perfume, and accessories. The ability to listen and hold an intelligent conversation draws men to her like moths to flame. Skills such as dancing, singing, writing, or playing a musical instrument enhance desirability.

All spruced up, the man meets his likewise ready, bejewelled ladylove with flowers in her flowing hair. But where does he take her? Vatsyayana stressed the setting of the rendezvous—a secluded, clean, sweet-smelling room with a canopied bed, pillows, and bolsters. Fruit or sweetmeats of her preference, a board game, a musical instrument, or a book of poetry completes the ambience. Rooms should ideally open into a garden with fragrant flowers and birdsong and include a swing or a bench in a bower. While most of us lack such an ideal environment, ensuring privacy in a clean room with a proper bed, firm pillows, and perhaps some music or poetry is achievable. Embellishing the space with flowers and perfume signals to a woman that she is treated as a person, not an object, making her more receptive to his overtures.

The next step should be an unhurried dalliance: The sweet agony of postponed fulfilment is as pleasurable as the act itself. The man should test the waters; if she does not resist, or feigns resistance for him to overcome, he should proceed gradually, moving from subtle to more pressing overtures until he can see in her eyes that she is ready for union. Postponing beyond this point signifies an unaccomplished lover.

At times, she may resist despite her liking for the man and the ambience. Even if he is aroused, he must stop, for she is not ready. No matter how frustrating, he should neither force nor hurry her, but escort her home without resentment. Her reticence may reflect inhibitions or timidity; she simply needs more time. If she returns willingly the next day, he may plant a gentle kiss. If she responds but pulls away, she requires further thawing. His restraint will ultimately win her over.

As for newlyweds, most couples in our country, even now, are strangers to each other. On their wedding night, it is unwise for a man to force himself on his new wife without easing her into intimacy. He should take at least four days to consummate the marriage. Initially, he can hold lengthy conversations, embrace only her upper body, kiss her gently, and brush lightly across her nipples. As he gains her confidence over, on subsequent nights, he can caress her thighs, kiss deeply, and, if she does not object, gradually proceed downwards to mutual delight. By the fourth night, he may consummate the marriage with finesse and consideration. Historically, boys of marriageable age were sent to courtesans to hone their skills in the art of love.

Vatsyayana also categorised men and women according to anatomical dimensions, advising that individuals with matching proportions should mate. Hence, a 'horse' man (longest penis) should pair with an 'elephant' woman (deepest vagina), a 'bull' with a 'mare', and a 'hare' with the smallest 'deer' woman.

More than the size of the organ, what matters to a woman is the staying power of the man, for Vatsyayana knew that women take a longer time to climax; hence the need for the man to be long-timed. If he is not, he should bring her to such levels of preparedness during foreplay that she is ready to climax when the act begins. He also observed that a man climaxes quickly the first time but takes longer during subsequent sessions in the same night, whereas the opposite holds true for a woman—she takes longer to climax the first time but attains orgasm more quickly during later unions.

Regarding the actual physicality of the act, Vatsyayana begins with the embrace and the kiss, which may occur simultaneously or sequentially. He classifies the embrace into four categories, each with myriad variations. The first two types of embraces are for those attracted to each other but have not yet spoken. The man may pass close to the woman, 'inadvertently' brushing against her body. If she does not object, they may take their dalliance to the next level. At times, the woman may take the initiative, pretending to pick something from the floor so that her cleavage is in full view. He could pull her close and hold her tight. Those who have declared their attraction may rub their bodies against each other while walking in the dark, or the man may press her against a wall or pillar. When they finally engage in intercourse, the woman may cling to him like a vine, put one foot on his, press against his thighs, wind the other leg around him, moaning all the while, cup his face, and draw his head down for a kiss. Returning to the embrace, the couple may shift from vertical to horizontal while still clinging to each other. The sage had names for different types of embraces. For instance, the one in which lovers almost merge into one another is called 'the mixture of milk and water'.

As for kissing, he stresses that it is not merely the meeting of lips. The lover may begin by kissing her hair, eyes, mouth, neck, or breasts. Genitalia should not be kissed at this time, as it would be 'too much, too early'. There are numerous ways of kissing: He may press her lips with his, rub his lips over hers at a slant, take both her lips in his, alternate upper and lower lips, or create a tunnel with his thumb and finger to glide his tongue in, press it against her teeth, sweep it over her palate, or duel with her tongue. The lovers may, in playful jousts, wager over who will get hold of the other's lower lip first. The man may let her win at first and beg for another round; if she loses, she may 'cheat' and take his lower lip in hers while he feigns sleep, setting the mood for another exciting session.

The guru is not averse to the use of gentle marks of passion—bites or nail impressions—provided they are consensual. Some may be aroused by it, while others are not, and the partner's preference must always be respected. If the pain enhances pleasure, by all means continue, but if it is distasteful or hurts, stop. Marks are made as keepsakes, reminders of passion, so one may relive and enjoy it later when alone. Nails should be clean and healthy, and teeth evenly set and sharp. However, a man should not leave visible marks on another's wife, or on a woman averse to such foreplay, for obvious reasons.

If, despite the elaborate preamble, the woman is still not ready, he may use his fingers to moisten and soften her vagina. Regarding intercourse itself, Vatsyayana says that although a man has only one lingam and a woman only one yoni, the ways in which they may unite are manifold. Monotony kills passion, and variety—whether in seduction, setting, or position—keeps it alive. The couple must be ready to experiment and give full rein to their imagination. Even in the missionary position, the man may thrust gently or firmly, upwards, downwards, sideways against one vaginal wall and then the other, or rotate his organ inside. The woman is an active participant, adopting various positions to accommodate the pulsing male organ. Positions include widely open, clasping, rising, split bamboo, crab, lotus, all-fours ('cow'), sitting, reclining, standing against a wall, or entwining her legs around him. Most men enjoy positions with the woman on top, raising and lowering or churning her hips.

Vatsyayana describes sixty-four methods of uniting male and female organs, achievable only by the most flexible and devoted lovers, though mastery is not required for enjoyment. The important thing is that both partners enjoy the act and monotony does not set in.

According to Vatsyayana, nothing in sex is taboo if mutually acceptable. Group sex—one woman with multiple men, as practiced in some hilly districts—was permitted, either individually or simultaneously. Women in harems could also engage with a man if fortune allowed.

The master was clearly not a prude. He even advocated oral sex, despite its taboo status in his time. Religious restrictions did not concern him. He endorsed the 'kakila' position (sex in the manner of crows), known today as '69', allowing both partners oral access simultaneously. He also allowed the use of an artificial penis or mechanical device for sexual enjoyment, provided it did not harm or involve the killing of a living being.

Perhaps most surprisingly, Vatsyayana taught men how to seduce another's wife in a section titled '*Paradarika*'. Feelings of guilt, shame, or sin should not mar the supreme ecstasy, which he likened to oneness with God. What concerned him was not morality but the practical consequences of the action. A man should pursue a married woman only if his love for her is intense enough to affect his sanity or will to live. Married women who dislike their husbands, whose husbands travel extensively, or whose husbands insult them or are below them in rank or ability, may be receptive to an extramarital affair. Equally important is knowing when to withdraw if the woman cools off. Stalking, blackmail, or other vengeful activities are explicitly discouraged.

If Vatsyayana were alive today, women worldwide would kiss his feet in gratitude. He educated men about female pleasure and, most importantly, the etiquette of a thoughtful denouement. In *Kama Sutra: The Art of Making Love to a Woman,* Pavan K. Varma notes that Vatsyayana advised: 'A good lover should have the refinement to bring physical intimacy to an aesthetic finale. He should make her feel wanted and loved, so she knows he is not in it only for sex. He could hold her close, stroke her hair, murmur sweet nothings in her ear, or conduct a loving, meaningful conversation . . . the post-coital cocoon of relaxed intimacy created by a thoughtful man can be a source of unique pleasure.'

Centuries ago, post-coital tenderness was considered the most satisfying part of intimacy. Modern men often fail here, turning over and sleeping, or leaving after clandestine encounters—creating a void in a woman's heart, arms, and bed. Regardless of marital status, the man must treat a woman with love and respect. The guru reiterates that female enjoyment and climax are paramount, as is treating her as a person, not a sexual object.

I do wish men and women all over the world go through this wonderful treatise that India has given to the world, the basic tenet of which is female pleasure and satisfaction that lays the foundation of a sound marriage or a good relationship. A fact that most tend to overlook. It also lays emphasis on the fact that innovation and variety are essential to sustaining passion; monotony takes the joy out of intimacy. Also, a man who hesitates too long, even when the woman is ready, is an incompetent lover. As we have seen, there are just three points to remember if one wants to enjoy a lifetime of ecstasy.

18

Tantric Sex

I would like to confess that much of my knowledge on the subject comes from the book *Tantra: The Secret Power of Sex* by Arvind and Shanta Kale. Like most people, I, too, was wary of Tantrics and their seemingly bizarre customs: Living in cremation grounds, smearing ash from funeral pyres on their foreheads, the use of skulls, worship of menstrual blood, consuming the flesh of burning bodies, and unusual sexual practices. Tantrics personified everything that an ordinary person might fear or abhor. The above-mentioned book opened my eyes to a whole new world, one where sexual union was unity with God, a oneness attained by the ascetic through abstinence, by the yogi through meditation, and by the dervish through ecstatic dance and swoons.

Tantra existed 2,500 years before the birth of Christ and was widely practised until puritans took control of the region and forced it into hiding. It is a comprehensive system that embraces emotions, the psyche, the subconscious, the middle conscious, and the conscious mind. The special qualities of these levels are honed and used.

Tantra believes in the duality of all things on earth; everything, animate or inanimate, is either male or female, nothing in between. It relies heavily on sexuality because 'in the beginning of all creation, Shiva and Shakti were united in such complete bliss that they could not distinguish themselves and thought of themselves only as Shiva. Then Shakti opened her eyes and became aware of herself as a separate identity, though she was still locked in ecstatic intercourse with Shiva. At the next stage, they were no longer connected in intercourse, but the chains of desire bound them to each other.'

The mere repetition of the sexual act, with as many women as possible and as many times in a day, is not the Tantric way, though the West often seems to believe it is the ultimate sexual experience. When the British first came to India, their soldiers boasted of their sexual prowess, though bazaar sex workers called them 'sparrows' for their brief, meaningless copulations. Even the legendary lovers of the West, Casanova and Don Juan, would have been held in contempt by Tantric masters, for Tantric sex is prolonged sex.

The first victim of the fast-paced life and energy-draining careers in the modern world is a person's sex life. The Western rush to tear off clothes, the haste to finish, and the glorification of quick orgasms, as seen in movies, are definitely not the Tantric way. The faster an orgasm is achieved, or the more times a man copulates with multiple women, the more glorified he is in the Western view. For women, the more willing she is to forgo the delights of foreplay, the more ready she is for penetrative sex, and the quicker she reaches orgasm, or fakes it, the more 'in demand' she is considered. Sexual acts such as oral sex squeezed into a lunch break or hurried adulterous encounters in a closet while a spouse reads the newspaper upstairs are often celebrated as daringly erotic.

The symbol of Tantra is the erect phallus in a receptive yoni before orgasm, for the staying power of a Tantric is seldom less than forty-five minutes. One of the most rewarding aspects of Tantra is maintaining sexual tension between partners for prolonged periods, with a constant sexual partner of similar maturity. Though Tantrics believe both men and women are polygamous, the intensity of the sexual experience that a pair of Tantric lovers painstakingly master together after innumerable hours of practice is so strong that they seldom feel the need to change partners for variety.

Tantra delights in the dissimilarity between the sexes, for 'the greater the sexual attributes are polarised, the greater will be the power generated when both sexes merge'. Making love the Tantric way is time-consuming and requires elaborate preparation: Body hygiene, erotic sartorial choices, physical fitness, and a well-equipped Tantric room.

Odours

There is no question that scent plays an important role in sexual attraction, though humans are not as overt as dogs in sniffing. Added to this is the taste of a lover's skin, which combines to create a heady flavour. Personal odour is created mainly by sweat glands, concentrated in the underarms and pubic area, combined with other bodily scents. If sweat is trapped for prolonged periods in hairy body parts or under thick clothing, bacteria grow and produce offensive odour. To avoid this, Tantrics strongly recommend the removal of body hair. Oral hygiene is also paramount.

The scent of the genitalia contributes to sexual attraction. Prostatic fluid imparts its distinctive odour to semen, while female sexual organs emit a scent that strongly attracts the male. Bartholin's glands, located on either side of the vaginal opening, secrete a scented fluid during sexual excitement for lubrication. This is augmented by vaginal secretions and the mucous plug at the cervix that is expelled during arousal. Menstrual fluid has a distinctive odour that excites some men. Natural body odours are not inherently repulsive, though the subtle use of perfume can enhance the sexual experience.

Exercise

As Tantric sex is sustained sex, it is energy-consuming and requires a high level of physical fitness. A single act of sex, as commonly practised, increases heart rate, respiration, and blood pressure to a significant degree in just sixty seconds. A healthy adult can manage this surge for a short time, but one must be truly fit to sustain it for the prolonged periods that Tantric sex entails. Hence, the importance of regular physical exercise, like Hatha Yoga. These exercises are not strenuous but aim to increase flexibility, strengthen core muscles, and control the specialised muscles of the genital region. Practising them with a partner makes them more enjoyable.

Dress

Dress should be provocative, for nudity alone is not inherently erotic, as anyone living in nudist camps can attest. Herein lies the need for erotic attire. Basic to a Tantric woman's wardrobe are three flimsy dupattas, black, red, and white, which may be draped to tantalising effect, hiding the breasts and sex organs while leaving other areas exposed. A single loose knot at the back of the neck allows the garment to be removed easily. Beads threaded on strong nylon may also be used to cover sexual parts.

Erotic lingerie is essential. It may include bras with cut-out nipple areas or pasties, cholis with large holes exposing the breasts, thongs, flimsy panties, or bloomers with a slit in the genital area, visible only when the thighs are parted. Men may wear loincloths outlining their genitals, tight Lycra breeches, or loose lungis or pyjamas, through which an erection is visibly evident.

Now that the basics have been attended to, the stage has to be set in the Tantric room, which should have four essentials: Seclusion, a beautiful view, a garden not visible to prying eyes, and a bathroom with a sunken tub fitted with railings. There should be mirrors everywhere, dim lighting, soft music, an erotic library, and videos of the couple making love, which can be a great turn-on.

The room should be well ventilated, for there is increased consumption of oxygen during prolonged copulation. It should also be soundproof, for uninhibited sex involves a great deal of noise. This is a tall order indeed, and not possible for most who live in small modern flats with parents and children in adjoining rooms. Such couples can keep the bedroom in the far corner for themselves and convert their balcony into a garden, perhaps covering it with creepers so that it is not accessible to prying eyes. The door should have a lock and a curtain, lest someone peep in through the keyhole. If noises from the kitchen or children intrude, they should reserve sexual activities for quiet afternoons or nights. Children should be made to understand that they are not to disturb their parents during 'meditation' or 'yoga'. Tantrics do take their sexuality seriously, and why not? It is among the most pleasurable activities known to humankind and, unlike animals, the human female does not have a restricted mating cycle.

As for the bed, it should be the regular rectangular type, though the height should be such that the man does not have to crouch, stand on tiptoe, or put cushions under the woman while making love with the man standing. It should have a single double-bed mattress, as twin mattresses tend to part during Tantric sex, cotton pillows that can be moulded according to need, and a bolster to support the back. A good floor rug that does not slip is essential, as is an armless chair with a broad base and a high, broad back.

Tantrics believe in social intercourse before sexual intercourse: Conversing, eating light snacks, and drinking mellowed wine in moderation to loosen inhibitions and delay the orgasmic response. This should be followed by light, fluttering kisses. The couple should spend at least an hour kissing on the mouth, with no other parts of their bodies touching. This defers orgasm and gives great sensuous pleasure, though the engorged sex organs clamour for release. In such a situation, they should let go and come up for air.

The man should then gradually move downward, kissing her neck, her cleavage, and the fullness of her breasts all around, occasionally holding the area around the nipples between his lips and breathing warmly on them. This will make them hard and erect, and the woman will long for her partner to suck these erect, yearning peaks, but he should refrain. Instead, he should breathe warmly on them and lick them. Only after this should he hold each breast firmly in turn between his lips and suck briefly. The sounds made during foreplay are erotic, and there should be no inhibitions on that score. This includes a liberal use of explicit language, which can be a powerful stimulus.

At this point, the man should pause his erotic stimulation and stroke her gently to cool her down. After stroking her forehead, ears, eyes, cheeks, lips, and throat, taking in the head and the nape of the neck in the final sweeping stroke, he should kiss each part gently and then begin the process all over again.

The man's attention will now be centred on the breasts, which are best stimulated by a natural milking action. He should lie at right angles to her and squeeze both breasts with both hands at the same time, gently at first, gradually increasing the pressure and moving his hands towards the nipples as if drawing milk from them. The nipples may then be pinched, rolled between thumb and forefinger, or held between the index and middle finger, as if holding a cigarette, and lightly scratched with the nail of the thumb, which gives intense pleasure to some women. This should be interlaced with intermittent sucking, depending on what the woman enjoys most. All this while, the woman may caress his face, head, and upper body, though she should not make contact with the penis, even if its rigidity aches for attention.

The man now lightly strokes her back, buttocks, stomach, thighs, and legs, drawing attention away from the highly erotic breast fondling in order to decrease her level of arousal and thereby prolong their intercourse. He can draw his finger along her inner thigh, over the vulval slit, and onto her stomach, while stroking other parts of her body with his other hand. He should then casually let his arm fall between the woman's legs, which she would have parted by now, and, on the upward movement, let his fingers glide into her genital lips but not into her vagina.

He then touches the clitoris gently with the ball of his index finger, with nails clipped short. He can roll it between his fingers, stroke it up and down, and excite the tip delicately, lubricating it, if necessary, with her vaginal secretions. At this stage, the woman should lightly stroke, not grasp, the penis. This releases the sexual pressure of the man somewhat instead of enhancing it. The stroking should be restricted to the upper part of the penis only, starting from the head to the base and then from the base to the head. She should not touch the undersurface or encircle it at this time. Only when the male organ is filmed with pre-coital fluid should they, at long last, begin intercourse.

This, too, must be done in a graded manner to prolong the duration of pleasure after insertion, for this is but the beginning of the next level of ecstasy and not the culmination of the prolonged foreplay. The semi-lateral position is best suited for this. The man lies in a semi-recumbent position, the upper part of his body supine, while the prone upper part of the woman lies upon him, their lower limbs entwined in a lateral position. The head of the man's penis is now enclosed in the moist socket at the junction of the genital lips, where the clitoris lies. This again acts as a restraint, for direct entry of the thrusting penis into the welcoming vagina may result in immediate release, thus negating all that they have sought to achieve.

When, after five to ten minutes, the urge for intromission subsides, the penis should be inserted into the vagina, but only to a depth of about three centimetres. This is an extremely difficult discipline, for both partners will wish to culminate the prolonged sexual tension, but control is the essence of a true Tantric. Deep breathing for two minutes may help, after which the man withdraws and places the head of his organ at the vulva.

The next time, insertion is to half the length of the penis, and the in-and-out movements should be slow and deliberate, each lasting for three minutes. Every fourth insertion should be complete but slow, after which every third and then every second insertion should be full, and the act is culminated as described above.

During the entire session, there may be graceful shifts from the semi-lateral position to the woman on top. Pelvic floor exercises have trained them amply to enhance sexual pleasure: The man to raise and lower his penis by tightening and relaxing his buttocks, while the woman can contract and relax her vaginal muscles, raise herself up and down, or make rotatory movements.

If, even after all this, orgasmic control is still maintained, they may switch to the rear-entry position, both lying on their sides facing the same direction, their bodies forming a 'V' bent at the genital region. In this position, he can caress her breasts with his lower arm and stimulate her clitoris with the upper one, which exquisitely heightens erotic sensation. Though the penis is completely inside, no movements should be made, allowing further control. In any case, movements are restricted by this position. This process of semi-insertion and withdrawal continues for about fifteen minutes, after which it is time to complete the act. The man makes shallow, rapid strokes until he feels the woman clasp him tightly, after which he thrusts deep and hard for an orgasmic ecstasy that the couple may never have experienced before.

They may also make use of the bathtub with railings all around, as the buoyancy of water gives an added boost, and try a host of other positions, such as sitting or standing, which are beyond the purview of this book. As it is, in these days of haste, presentations, deadlines, sleep deprivation, and perpetual fatigue, one wonders how many of us will have the inclination, patience, and passion to indulge in such prolonged sex, though the rewards are many, not the least of which is a deep and enduring bond with one's partner.

19

The Perfumed Garden

Mohammed, the Prophet, discussed sexual intercourse and marriage in the Qur'an. The Muslim is directed to marvel at the process of procreation, which is second only to the creation of heaven and earth. It was considered a religious act. Breastfeeding was advocated until the child was two years old, and rightly so, while incest, sleeping with one's wife's sister, a married woman, prostitutes, and women deemed morally corrupt were forbidden. The Prophet had twenty-one wives, and it was believed that one could have sexual relations with two at a time, and he advised his followers to 'marry whom you please'. Divorce was permitted, and a widow could remarry three months and ten days after her husband's death.

Sheikh Nefzaoui writes:

> Praise be given to God who has placed man's greatest pleasure in the natural parts of woman and has destined the natural parts of man to afford the greatest enjoyment for woman.
>
> He has not endowed the parts of woman with any pleasurable or satisfactory feeling until they have been penetrated by the instrument of the male; and likewise, the sexual organs of the male know neither rest nor quietness until they have entered those of the female.

The Arabs had a penchant for chubby women, for besides her eyes with 'lashes like polished blades', her rounded cheeks and ample breasts, they found her double chin and the rolls of flesh on her belly, with its deep navel, very seductive. Had the modern Arab not been influenced by Western ideals, plus-sized women from the West might have gone there in droves to reclaim their self-esteem, desired for the very flesh that repulsed the Western man. Even prehistoric men preferred women with fat on their bellies, thighs, and buttocks, and with good reason. These reserves would nourish his child in her womb during times of scarcity.

With her swelling breasts and majestic crupper, God has bestowed upon woman an 'empire of seduction'. Her pudenda, described as the 'arena of combat', is lavishly eulogised in the book. According to the Sheikh, it has a mouth and a tongue, the clitoris, and resembles the impression of a gazelle's hoof on desert sands, but when endowed with ample flesh, it is likened to the head of a lion. 'Oh! How many men's deaths lie at her door!'

They even classified different types of vulva, ranging from El Feurdj (the slit), the voluptuous, the beautiful, the duellist, the humpbacked (with a high mount of Venus), the one ever ready for the fray, the sucker, the delicious, the crusher, and the fiery one. Least desirable were the hedgehog, the vulva of a decrepit old woman dried up with age and bristly hair, and the juicy one, considered the most repulsive of all for the abundance of secretions that appear even with the man's initial caresses and are thought to repel him. There were, of course, classifications of the male organ as well, ranging from the extinguisher of passion, the house-breaker, and the indomitable, which were greatly preferred by women, to the pigeon, the flabby one, and the weepy one.

Dreams of the vulva and of coition were believed to have various interpretations. It was considered auspicious to dream of an open vulva, which brought prosperity and freedom from troubles, while the closed vulva of a virgin indicated that doors would not open and desires would not be fulfilled. Dreaming of a man copulating with a woman and seeing her vulva after he disengages was said to bring a fruitful conclusion to a business venture with that man's help. If the dreamer sees himself mounted on a woman and later sees her private parts, he would obtain success through his own efforts. If a man begins intercourse in his dream but does not complete the act, he would meet with failure in his ventures. This gives a whole new meaning to dream interpretation centuries before Freud.

The Sheikh goes on to say that men prefer women who are sweet-smelling, plump, and lusty. As for the behaviour of the ideal woman, she should cover herself adequately and remain within the home. She should laugh and speak rarely, not complain or cry, have no female friends, and confide solely in her husband. She should accept gifts only from her husband and parents. If her husband desires sex, she should agree to it and even provoke it at times. She must not give in to carnal desires with anyone else, even if abstinence were to cause her suffering. A tall order indeed.

As for the attributes of a praiseworthy man, he should be good-looking but not conceited, should respond sexually on finding himself near a woman, and must be eager to please her. He should fill her vagina completely and ejaculate after prolonged coitus to give sustained pleasure. The act itself is likened to the pounding of a pestle in a mortar. After release, he should soon be ready again, for the woman is said to value the man primarily for sexual fulfilment. Most important of all, he should not boast of his conquests. Even today, a man who kisses and tells is abhorred by cultures across the world.

Sex should be avoided on a full stomach, as it is difficult to perform vigorously soon after a meal. Moreover, no woman would appreciate a belch in her face during the act. Though paederasty was prevalent among some communities at the time, indulgence in anal or oral sex with a woman was frowned upon.

The very name *The Perfumed Garden* bears testimony to the importance of scent in sexual attraction, and to the belief that perfume arouses desire in both sexes. Inhaling a man's perfume could send a woman into a swoon and assist him in possessing her. Prophet Mohammed's rival, Mocailama the impostor from the tribe of Honicifa, used this knowledge to seduce the prophetess Chedja et Temimia of the Beni-Temim tribe. She became his rival after the Prophet's death and declared that prophecy could not belong to two persons. Either he was the prophet, in which case she and her disciples would follow his laws, or she was the prophetess and he and his followers would follow hers. She sent him an ultimatum, adding that she was coming with her followers to determine who that one would be. Mocailama consulted his aide, who advised him to erect a brocade tent outside the city, fill it with silk furnishings and perfumes of every variety, musk, rose, orange blossom, hyacinth, carnation, jasmine, including those released when burned on coals, such as amber. He was to sit on his throne and beckon her inside only when the vapour was strong enough to scent even water.

When the prophetess entered the tent, she was overcome by sensual desire. Pressing his advantage, Mocailama asked her which position she preferred: On her back, on all fours, bent forward, or on her knees like a tripod, as in prayer. In this posture, the posterior is thrust upwards and backwards, making the crupper easily accessible. She desired all of them. Soon after, the two were married. Such was the aphrodisiac power of perfumes as understood by the ancients centuries ago. It remains true even today, though one may be sceptical of advertisements showing women abandoning everything to follow a man after a single whiff.

Excerpts from various parts of the book emphasise that pleasure should be equal and mutual. Just as the basil plant releases its scent only when its leaves are rubbed, so it is with a woman. Only after kissing, nibbling, and caressing her can one obtain what one desires by awakening affection and longing. Only when her lips tremble, her eyes grow dreamy, and her sighs quicken should he enter her for a coitus satisfying to both. Stress is laid on both partners reaching orgasm simultaneously, for he will then feel her vagina clasp his penis, resulting in exquisite pleasure. The Sheikh also advises that the man should not rise immediately after the act, but withdraw gradually and remain close to the woman, lying on her right side. A man who removes himself abruptly and rises, like an unrefined animal, robs a woman of all pleasure. *How true!*

Besides the innumerable positions that a healthy couple of average height and build could adopt to enhance pleasure, others were suggested for special circumstances. For instance, a man with a short penis could have the woman assume the posture adopted during prayer or lie supine with her legs raised straight to her ears, one on each side of her head, so that her private parts protrude and he has easy access. The book also mentions positions for the obese, whether one or both partners, and for those with physical deformities, so that no one is deprived of sexual pleasure.

While writing about these various positions, I was proud to read that the Sheikh acknowledged India as being far advanced in such matters and that many coital positions were learnt from us. I wonder where that India has gone.

Part IV

Challenges in Female Sexual Health

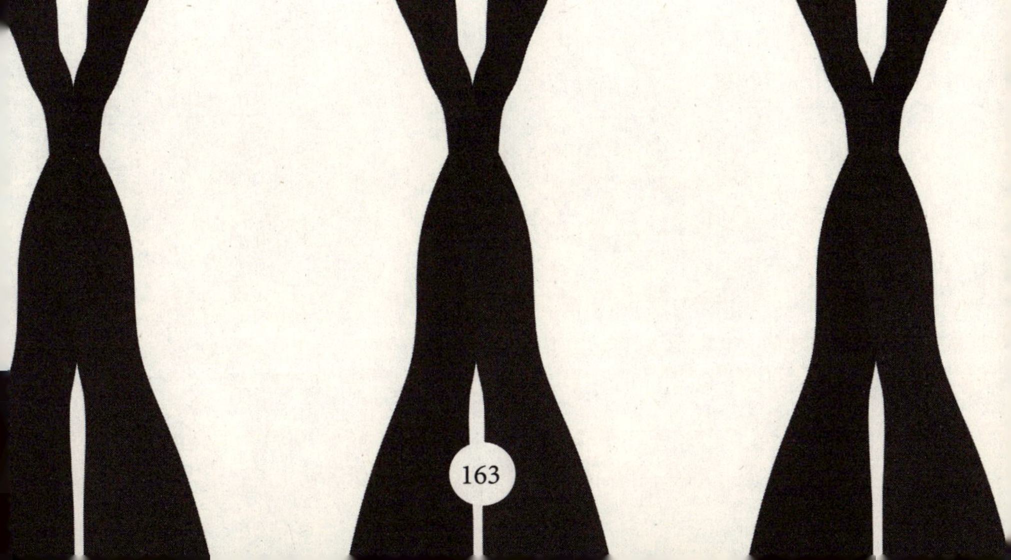

20

Sexual Dysfunction

It would not be out of place to explain the meaning of sexual health before we elaborate on the various types of sexual dysfunction that can occur. The World Health Organization (WHO) defines sexual health as a state of physical, mental, and social well-being in relation to sexuality.

Most issues arising in a marriage or relationship can be traced to incompatibility in bed. Conversely, no matter how serious a disagreement between partners, a thorough, satisfying session in bed smooths out the differences, placing the relationship back on track. Sadly, this is not always the case. The 'fault', if one may call it so, could be in the man, like difficulty in attaining or sustaining an erection or premature ejaculation. More often than not, it is the lack of knowledge or expertise in the technique of foreplay and female arousal that needs to be addressed for a satisfying sex life.

On the other hand, we have a bunch of female sexual disorders that can be grouped under 'Female Sexual Dysfunction (FSD)' that involve persistent or recurrent issues with desire, arousal, orgasm, or pain during the sexual act, which will be discussed in the following chapters.

A woman in great distress came to me one day. She was the second wife of a man who compared her unfavourably with his first wife. As a result, her self-esteem had plummeted to dismal depths. What hurt her most was that he thought she was 'cold' in bed, while the first wife had been passionate. She would come back from a ladies' sangeet so charged with sexual energy that she would wake him up to satiate her desire; ever eager for sex, she liked to be on top.

'And you lie limp beneath me like a rag doll,' he told her the day before, then got off her in disgust without completing the act.

'What should I do, doctor?' she wailed, bursting into tears. After some consolatory words and a glass of water, her story came tumbling out.

'I was brought up in a conservative household, and I do not know a thing about sex. In college, I fell in love with a classmate, but we went no further than exchanging love notes. I wanted to marry him, but with four daughters, my father thought it best to marry me off to this widower with two children just because he wanted no dowry. That I needed to be initiated gently in bed did not occur to this brute, who now blames me for our unsatisfactory sex life. I spend the entire day playing nanny, housekeeper, cook, and maid, without rest or respite. That the house is well kept and the children well looked after does not earn me a word of appreciation. Tired to the bone, I lie on the bed only to be used and then told that I am no good. Though my skin crawls at his touch and his taunts hurt like whiplashes, I see no way out of this hopeless situation.'

God knows she had enough reasons to be unresponsive to this man—lack of attraction, foreplay, rest, and appreciation were enough to kill desire in any woman, more so in one in whom it had not been awakened at all. To compare her unfavourably with a deceased wife was the worst thing he could do. Added to this was blaming her for lacking ardour when he was the culprit all along. Like most men, he could never believe that the fault lay with him.

Then there was a neighbour, married to a man whose business took him on tours. He would be away for days and expect a rousing welcome on his return but found her to be 'cold and unresponsive', which put him off. Hurt and angry, she told him one day, 'You should be glad that you do not have a passionate wife. With you away for most of the month, I might have taken a lover and foisted his child on you, or run away with another.'

Though he agreed with her logic, he would have liked a more interested bed partner so that their union was not a joyless necessity for him and a chore for her.

Were these two women truly 'frigid'? If so, what does that term mean, and can the condition be treated? These are some of the questions addressed in this chapter.

Frigidity, a dated and pejorative term, was traditionally used to describe a woman's failure to respond to sexual stimuli. The word is derived from the Latin *frigidus* (cold), with the suffix *-ity* from *-itas* (state). Today, this issue is more appropriately grouped under the umbrella of Female Sexual Dysfunction (FSD), defined as persistent or recurrent problems with sexual desire, arousal, orgasm, or pain that cause distress to the woman or strain her relationship with her partner.

FSD may occur at any age and at any phase of the sexual response cycle—excitement, plateau, orgasm, or resolution—and can prevent a woman from experiencing sexual satisfaction. She may have little or no desire for sex, be unable to become aroused despite adequate stimulation, be sufficiently aroused but unable to achieve orgasm, or experience pain during intercourse. The causes may be hormonal or psychological, or there may be a physical basis for painful intercourse.

Psychological factors contributing to FSD include stress, anxiety, depression, fatigue, worry, guilt, trauma, abuse, relationship difficulties, boredom with routine sex, an undesirable partner or setting, poor body image, fear of pregnancy, or concerns about sexual performance. Vaginismus, an involuntary spasm of the muscles around the vaginal opening, can prevent penetration despite the absence of any physical abnormality.

Physical factors include pain during intercourse, alcohol or substance misuse, hormonal fluctuations during pregnancy and after childbirth, diabetes, cardiac, renal, hepatic, or neurological disease, certain medications, ageing, and menopause.

Female sexual dysfunction may present as:

1. **Lack of Sexual Desire:** Arising from any of the psychological or physical issues mentioned above. Lifestyle changes such as adequate rest, relief from drudgery and childcare, or an out-of-station holiday with a supportive partner can help rekindle desire in a harried housewife or a woman with a stressful job. Reviewing medications that affect libido and treating conditions such as depression or chronic illness may also help reclaim one's sex life. A change of routine—trying new positions, settings, or times of day, even incorporating consensual fantasy or role play—may further help reignite sexual desire.
2. **Inability to Become Aroused:** It may occur when the partner does not engage in sufficient foreplay or fails to stimulate specific erogenous zones. The timing or situation may not be conducive to sex, or there may be boredom arising from routine. Insufficient vaginal lubrication can also be a cause, especially in ageing women due to an anticipatory dread of pain.
3. **Anorgasmia:** Some women are unable to achieve orgasm, no matter how caring their partner may be. The reasons can range from relationship difficulties and inadequate arousal techniques to stress, fatigue, poor physical or mental health, gynaecological conditions such as pelvic pain or sexually transmitted infections, or a history of sexual trauma.

Management of Female Sexual Dysfunction

Communication is key. Understanding with one's partner should be nurtured to the extent that a woman can express what feels pleasurable and what does not—or better still, guide him to her erogenous zones. She may teach him how to use his hands or mouth in a way that feels right to her. Such openness can be difficult for a woman brought up in a conservative household where discussions around sex were taboo. It requires patience and sensitivity on the part of a loving partner to draw her out, but if he succeeds, both stand to gain immensely.

If this proves difficult, the couple may aim for non-coital intimacy, which can help alleviate performance anxiety. It can be deeply comforting to curl up and sleep in a partner's embrace without the pressure of sexual performance or the guilt of disappointing him weighing on her mind. Listening to music or watching television or videos together can also be pleasurable non-coital activities that foster closeness. A sensual massage is another effective way of helping a woman relax and feel more comfortable with her partner, which may, in turn, enhance communication. Kegel exercises are beneficial in some cases as well.

If self-help measures do not work, or if the woman feels too embarrassed to express her desires openly, a visit to a doctor or sex therapist is warranted. The specialist will take a detailed history, including the woman's attitude towards sex, any history of sexual abuse, relationship issues, alcohol or substance use, chronic illnesses, medications, and a detailed obstetric history—particularly trauma or episiotomy during childbirth. The presence of the partner is advisable so that both can be counselled together. A thorough clinical examination will help confirm or rule out physical conditions contributing to sexual distress, which can then be treated appropriately. Vaginal dryness after menopause can often be managed effectively with lubricants and oestrogen creams.

Once underlying physical or psychological issues are addressed with professional help, most problems improve significantly. Of utmost importance is patient education. Familiarising a woman with normal anatomy, sexual responses, and the changes that occur during pregnancy and menopause can help ease her fears. It should be emphasised that she is entitled to enjoy sex, experiment, and live out her sexual fantasies. Sexual stimulation may be enhanced through guilt-free masturbation, rediscovering erogenous zones with a partner, changing sexual routines, or engaging with erotic literature or videos.

For women who previously experienced orgasms but have since become indifferent to sex, the cause may be boredom, fatigue, or routine. As mentioned earlier, trying different sexual positions, having sex at different times of the day, or in different settings can go a long way in rekindling desire. Sex can also be planned so that time and energy are conserved, allowing both partners to look forward to an unhurried encounter in a relaxed atmosphere.

Women experiencing pain during intercourse may benefit from changing positions that minimise or eliminate discomfort. Pain on entry may be due to vaginal dryness, fungal infections that cause small cuts at the vaginal opening, or a poorly healed episiotomy after delivery. While oestrogen creams help postmenopausal women, water-based lubricants can relieve pain caused by friction. Fungal infections can be treated with appropriate local or systemic medication, and a painful episiotomy can often be corrected with a minor surgical procedure. Pain during deep penetration is commonly due to endometriosis or pelvic inflammatory conditions, which may require medical or surgical treatment. In the meantime, the male partner should avoid deep thrusting; the woman may keep her legs straight during intercourse. Penile bumpers worn over an erect penis can also limit the depth of penetration. A non-steroidal anti-inflammatory drug (NSAID) taken prior to intercourse may reduce pain. Relaxation techniques, such as a warm bath or meditation before intercourse, can further decrease pain responses.

Hormones play a significant role in female sexual function. As women age, levels of the female sex hormone oestrogen decline, which can lead to reduced vaginal lubrication and decreased genital sensation. Low levels of testosterone—the hormone largely responsible for libido in women—may also contribute to reduced sexual arousal, diminished genital sensation, and anorgasmia. When not contraindicated, menopausal hormone therapy (MHT) may improve sexual function. Oestrogen helps combat urogenital atrophy, mood disturbances, and vasomotor symptoms such as hot flushes, all of which can negatively affect sexual well-being. MHT must be taken under strict medical supervision, as it is contraindicated in certain situations and requires regular follow-up. If vaginal dryness alone is the issue, lubricants or local vaginal oestrogen therapy are often sufficient.

A hysterectomy, the surgical removal of the uterus, may lead to reduced sexual responsiveness in up to 30 per cent of women. Nerves and blood vessels essential to sexual functioning may be affected during surgery. Removal of the ovaries causes a sudden and significant drop in female sex hormones, often resulting in loss of desire, decreased lubrication, and reduced genital sensation.[17]

Whether sexual dysfunction can be resolved depends largely on the underlying cause. When it is due to a treatable physical condition, the outcome is often favourable. When psychological factors are predominant, counselling and improved communication between partners can be highly effective. Many women experience a combination of contributing factors, all of which need to be addressed thoughtfully.

To summarise, sexual problems in women are relatively common, and nearly every woman may experience them at some point. If such problems persist or recur and cause distress to the woman or strain her relationship, seeking help is essential, for no woman should remain deprived of sexual pleasure, which is her rightful due.

21

Vaginismus

Here is a short story based on a real incident, which I wrote as part of my hugely popular series 'Diary of a Gynaecologist' for the widely read women's magazine *Woman's Era*. Before it was published, I had sent a copy to Khushwant Singh and was eagerly awaiting a response.

Rupali, as the name suggested, was beautiful. Slender, tall, and fair, her face had the radiance of the moon, on which an accomplished artist had sculpted the features of a woman. Her arms were supple stalks on which grew lily-white hands. Her eyes were dark brown, as was her hair, which hung in a loose plait down to her well-rounded hips. It was as if God had made her exclusively for love. The Zari-bordered red silk sari proclaimed her newly married status, as did the red and ivory *choora* on her wrists. She came to my clinic with her mother-in-law, who, besides her diamonds, wore an expression of barely concealed antagonism. The hostility was on account of the fact that Rupali had consistently denied her son his conjugal rights since their marriage a month back!

'Doctor,' said the portly matron, 'matters have progressed far beyond the traditional bashfulness of a new bride.' Her chest heaved in outrage, while Rupali gazed at me with the eyes of a stricken doe.

I took the terrified girl to the examination room and probed her gently. There was an angry red fissure in the hymenal region. The brute! He had forced himself upon her without finesse and was now adding insult to injury.

'The marriage has been consummated all right,' I informed the mother-in-law. 'The local area is still raw at the moment. I think it would be a good idea to send her to her parents' place till the wound heals.'

A month later, the situation had not improved. Rupali was a classic case of vaginismus, wherein a woman actively resists sexual intercourse, though there is nothing physically wrong with her. There was no history of sexual abuse; however, she feared sexual intercourse and actively resisted penetration. As she lay on the examination table with her knees bent and legs spread out, I smeared my gloved index finger liberally with a local anaesthetic jelly and gently inserted it into her vagina. She tightened up instantaneously and raised her buttocks with my finger still inside! Nothing I said would make her relax. This is what she did every time her husband tried to mount her.

'I am willing to stand between your legs the whole day with my finger cramped inside, if that's the way you want it,' I said calmly.

'I'm sorry, doctor, I'm so sorry, but I can't help myself,' she whimpered.

'You have nothing to fear. I have numbed the local area, and I'm sure you don't feel a thing.'

Gradually, it dawned upon her that she wasn't really hurting at all. It was purely a reflex action that led to this ludicrous stance. My perseverance paid and she relaxed. Now that I had gained her confidence, I inserted my second finger alongside the first. Again, the same response, but for a shorter period. An internal check-up revealed no abnormality.

She was genuinely concerned for her husband and felt miserable rejecting his advances night after night.

'Will blue films help?' she asked in desperation.

'I suggest that you read an authentic book on the subject.'

'Will that excite me?'

'Forget about getting excited at this point in time. Focus on getting to know your body. More importantly, let go of dread.'

'How do I do that?'

'Aim for a lack of sensations initially. Apply xylocaine jelly liberally and insert your own finger inside till you can tolerate it without tightening up.'

'Make sure that he uses a condom, for the local anaesthetic agent would numb his organ too, which will shrivel up.' I smiled, but she was not amused.

Not all appreciate my sense of humour. Moreover, it was ill-timed.

'But his organ is so thick!' she said innocently.

Ashamed of my frivolity, I resumed my professional manner and inserted a speculum inside her vagina to show her that there was space enough for his thick organ. An entire baby comes out of this very orifice.

'But what should I insert to make the opening larger?' asked the hapless girl.

As those were not the days of online shopping, and I was not aware of sex shops in India, I improvised and asked her to insert the sleek, slender variety of brinjal into her vagina after covering it with a condom.

A week later, a beaming Rupali returned with her handsome husband. It was the first time I met the person whose intimate life had been revealed to me on almost a daily basis. There was a glow about them, a shy happiness that told me all. It was gratifying to learn that one's treatment had succeeded. They put a box of sweetmeats on my table. This was indeed a first! I had often received sweets for delivering babies, but never for the consummation of a marriage! Even as I was pondering over this, Rupali took me aside and whispered in my ear.

'Doctor, the brinjal did not seem thick enough, so I used a carrot instead. I hope it's all right.'

I could barely contain my laughter till they left.

PS A fortnight later, Khushwant Singh called up to inform me that he had enjoyed the story immensely. Even as I beamed with the praise, he added, '*Tune tey gaajar, baigan de bha vadate* [You've increased the price of carrots and brinjals]!', which had us in splits.

⚥

Vaginismus refers broadly to involuntary muscle spasm that prevents the insertion of any object into the vagina, whether for sexual, medical, or hygienic purposes—including speculums or tampons. More specifically, it is characterised by involuntary contraction of the vaginal muscles that interferes with intercourse, even when the woman desires sexual intimacy. As with other female sexual dysfunctions, the diagnosis is made when symptoms cause significant personal distress.

Medically, vaginismus is defined as 'recurrent or persistent involuntary spasm of the musculature of the outer third of the vagina that interferes with sexual intercourse, causing marked distress or interpersonal difficulty.'

Approximately 0.5 per cent of women experience vaginismus. It is termed 'primary' when no physical abnormality is detected and symptoms appear when intercourse is first attempted. Contributing factors may include fear of pain, upbringing in environments that associate sex with shame, or feelings of aversion. Women with vaginismus are statistically more likely to report a history of childhood sexual abuse, although many cases have no identifiable cause.

'Secondary' vaginismus occurs in individuals who were previously able to achieve penetration but later developed symptoms. Common triggers include vaginal infections, endometriosis, childbirth-related trauma, surgical procedures, or vaginal dryness during the peri- or post-menopausal period.

Vaginismus is graded by severity:

- First degree—muscle spasm relieved by reassurance
- Second degree—spasm persists despite reassurance

- Third degree—elevation of the buttocks to avoid examination
- Fourth degree—retreat, elevation of the buttocks, and tight closure of the thighs
- Fifth degree—visceral reactions such as sweating, hyperventilation, palpitations, trembling, nausea, fainting, or extreme avoidance responses

Treatment options include lubrication, behavioural therapy, anxiolytics or antidepressants, pelvic floor physiotherapy, graduated exposure, and progressive vaginal dilatation. Botox injections are also being explored to relieve muscle spasm. A multidisciplinary approach, which combines the expertise of a gynaecologist, psychologist, sex therapist, and physical therapist, is often most effective. Outcomes vary, but patience, consistency, and reassurance remain central to successful treatment.

22

When Desire Becomes Compulsion

Down the ages, famous women—from Cleopatra and Catherine the Great to Napoleon's sister Pauline Bonaparte, Marie Antoinette, and present-day celebrities such as Angelina Jolie and Britney Spears—were labelled sex addicts or nymphomaniacs (the latter especially by 2000s tabloids and celebrity profiles). Much like a queen bee, Cleopatra was reputed to allow a man a single night with her on the condition that he would be executed the next day, and many reportedly agreed.

Beautiful Pauline was said to be involved in an incestuous relationship with her brother Napoleon, besides having numerous affairs with other men. As for Catherine the Great, there persists an enduring myth that she was crushed to death beneath a horse with which she was attempting to have sex. The truth is that she died of a stroke while seated on a toilet in her palace. She had around twenty lovers, whom she rewarded generously for their companionship. Some were even selected by a former lover with whom she remained friends after their relationship ended. If Catherine took a liking to a new man, his health was assessed by a physician and his sexual aptitude by her lady-in-waiting before he was introduced to her. It is another matter that when one lady-in-waiting continued her association with a chosen man even after he became the Empress's lover, she was exiled for life. Catherine chose not to remarry after her husband was overthrown and killed six months into his reign. Instead, she ruled Russia with remarkable success for thirty-four years. Like Elizabeth I of England, she did not wish to cede power to any man.

The beautiful Vivien Leigh—unforgettable as Scarlett O'Hara in *Gone with the Wind*—was often described as a sex addict, though in reality she was struggling with bipolar disorder, characterised by extreme highs and lows. It was during the manic phases that she indulged in excesses, including sexual ones. Our own Amrita Sher-Gil was similarly labelled a nymphomaniac and is believed to have been poisoned by a jealous husband, allegedly on account of her intense sexual appetite, which she expressed through multiple relationships.

Khushwant Singh once told me of a man who arrived at her home for their first rendezvous bearing flowers and champagne, only to find that this was not her style at all. The moment the door closed, she reportedly shed her clothes, lay down naked on the rug by the fire, and invited him to proceed without ceremony.

A self-described nymphomaniac once wrote on her blog that she needed at least five orgasms a day. To achieve this, she spent several hours pleasuring herself or having sex with men she picked up at supermarkets, until she eventually found her calling—testing sex toys for a company to determine what worked for women and what did not. Most women, unfortunately, are not fortunate enough to find a profession that aligns so closely with their desires.

What Is Hypersexuality?

Hypersexuality (also historically called Nymphomania) refers to excessive, uncontrollable sexual desire in a woman. She engages in repeated sexual behaviours without experiencing satisfaction and struggles unsuccessfully to restrain these urges. The term Nymphomania is derived from the Latin nymphae (the inner lips of the vulva) and *mania*. In Greek mythology, nymphs were depicted as sexually uninhibited female deities. Men with excessive sexual desire were historically described as suffering from *satyriasis*, named after satyrs—mythical male figures known for perpetual arousal and sexual pursuit.

In earlier times, physicians attempted to 'treat' nymphomania through practices that were not only misguided but brutal, including the removal of the clitoris. Menstruation was also believed to cause nymphomania, leading to the removal of ovaries—an intervention that may have reduced libido due to sudden hormone deprivation. Other so-called treatments included vaginal leeching, bloodletting, and application of cocaine to the vagina. When these failed, women were often confined to asylums.

Today, increased sexual desire in both men and women is described using the gender-neutral term 'hypersexuality'. It is also referred to as sexual addiction or compulsive sexual behaviour. While the WHO has included 'compulsive sexual behaviour' in the International Classification of Diseases, it is not categorised as a mental disorder.

So, how does one differentiate between a naturally high libido and sex addiction? It lies in the impact on daily functioning. A healthy sex drive does not interfere with day-to-day life, whereas sex addiction causes distress and impairment. The Mayo Clinic defines sexual addiction as 'an excessive preoccupation with sexual fantasies, urges, or behaviours that is difficult to control, causes distress, or negatively affects health, work, relationships, or other aspects of life'. Examples include compulsive masturbation, cybersex, multiple anonymous partners, or excessive use of pornography.

Risk factors include age under thirty, stress, family history of mental illness, same-sex orientation, personal psychiatric history, and recent traumatic life events. Although the precise cause remains unknown, contributing factors may be environmental, genetic, or related to chemical imbalances in the brain. Dormant tendencies may be triggered by life events. Symptoms include compulsive sexual behaviour, promiscuity, difficulty concentrating, feelings of shame, guilt, intrusive thoughts, and inability to control impulses. Consequences can include STIs, unwanted pregnancies, poor self-esteem, depression or anxiety, substance misuse, reduced productivity, relationship breakdowns, social withdrawal, and financial strain.

Medical intervention should be sought when harm outweighs pleasure. Warning signs include inability to control sexual impulses, emotional distress, impaired functioning, loss of employment, relationship breakdown, physical or legal complications, and thoughts of self-harm or suicide.

Treatment

Given the real risk of sexually transmitted infections and unintended pregnancies, compulsive sexual behaviour requires timely attention. Treatment approaches are similar to those used for obsessive–compulsive disorder and may include psychotherapy, cognitive behavioural therapy, family or social therapy, and medications such as anxiolytics, antidepressants, or antipsychotics. Self-management strategies include a balanced diet, regular exercise, adequate sleep, engagement in fulfilling non-sexual activities, social interaction, family support, and participation in support groups. Complementary therapies such as acupuncture, massage, yoga, and herbal remedies may also be beneficial.

A woman with compulsive sexual behaviour should never be shamed, ridiculed, or exploited. Her lack of control places her at significant risk of infection, unwanted pregnancy, and dangerous encounters. What she needs is understanding, family support, avoidance of known triggers, and appropriate medical and psychological care.

Then there are women with a healthy sexual appetite who are married to or are in a monogamous relationship with men with a low libido. How are they to quench their desire? Should they ask for more sex from a partner who is unable to provide it? It is a rare man who will understand and help her out with mutual masturbation or a greater emotional connection. Most take it as a slur on their manhood. As slaves to their egos, they end up using derogatory terms for her natural desires. Incensed beyond measure, one man sarcastically told his wife to sit in a brothel!

Though such barbs may take a subtler form in other households, the underlying sentiment remains the same. In a patriarchal society like ours, questioning a man's virility is tantamount to emasculation. What does she do then? The only two options available for her are self-gratification or an extramarital affair. Of the two, the former is safer and much less complicated. There should be no guilt attached to such activity. It will even out the temperature in an ice-and-fire marriage and restore harmony.

A young relative even brought her vibrator along when she came to spend a few days with me. When I expressed surprise, she told me, 'Why should I depend on a husband who is so busy at work that he is too tired for sex at night?

'This little companion of mine gives me more joy than he ever can. At least, I am not cheating on him!'

How true!

23

Genital Anatomy and Sexual Function

My life is anything but sweet, thought Madhu bitterly, wondering why her parents had named her Madhu, meaning honey. Only twenty years old, she had been married at sixteen and discarded at seventeen for being perceived as *hijra*, a term often used colloquially for intersex or gender-variant individuals. Though she had feminine contours and well-developed breasts, she had never menstruated. Assuming that some girls mature late, her mother concealed this fact from Madhu's in-laws, a decision that ultimately proved damaging.

Her year-long married life was marked by deep sexual frustration, despite her having normal sexual desire. Try as he might, her husband could not penetrate her. The persistent rubbing of his organ against her genitals aroused her, and after he fell asleep, she sought release through self-stimulation, only to be overwhelmed by guilt afterwards.

Her father abandoned her to her fate after her in-laws cast her out; he had neither the means nor the inclination to arrange another marriage or dowry. Madhu took up work as a full-time domestic help in a gynaecologist's household. The position provided her with food, shelter, and some money to spare. She also struck up a friendship with the gardener and his wife, who lived in the adjoining servant quarters, and would often play with their little son in her free time. Life, under the circumstances, was as good as it could be.

Madhu was a diligent worker, and her employer, Dr Manisha, was kind. Over time, they developed a friendship and began confiding in each other. When asked why her husband had left her, Madhu blurted out the painful story of her humiliating married life.

Dr Manisha grew pensive. The following day, she took Madhu with her to the government hospital where she worked and examined her thoroughly. Her suspicions were confirmed. Madhu did not have a vagina. An ultrasound revealed the absence of a uterus as well, although her ovaries were normal. Since the ovaries produced female sex hormones necessary for the development of secondary sexual characteristics, Madhu had normal breasts and body hair in the axillary and pubic regions. Without a uterus, she could neither menstruate nor conceive. As for the absent vagina, reconstructive surgery could create a neovagina capable of sexual function. Madhu, however, was reluctant to undergo the procedure, as she had no husband to share an intimate life with.

Then, one day, tragedy struck the household she had come to regard as her own. The gardener's wife died during childbirth, leaving behind a newborn daughter, a motherless toddler, and a grieving husband. Madhu helped as much as she could, but frequent visits to his home risked attracting gossip. She knew a sexual relationship was impossible, yet how was she to silence malicious tongues?

It was then that her kind employer suggested she marry the gardener. He readily agreed, and Madhu herself had developed affection for the gentle, burdened man. This time, she consented to the surgery Dr Manisha had earlier proposed. Along with a compassionate husband, she would gain children she had once believed she could never have. The surgery was successful, and after she had healed completely, the marriage was solemnised. Despite the hardships of her young life, Madhu finally found love and contentment in the servant quarters of her benevolent Doctor Madam's bungalow.

Most of us are unaware of such conditions, but it is sobering to acknowledge that nature, too, can falter. About 1 per cent of children born to the general population have congenital anomalies; this figure rises to 10 per cent or more in families with a history of birth defects. The risk also increases following certain infections, such as German measles, or exposure to specific medications during early pregnancy. Foetuses with anomalies incompatible with life do not survive till birth. Others, such as those with severe cardiac defects, may require surgery immediately after delivery, while milder malformations can be corrected later. Individuals with conditions that cannot be treated learn to live with them in an often-unforgiving world.

Since this book concerns female sexuality, it is important to note that a normally formed genital tract is essential for a normal sexual life. Although uncommon, congenital anomalies that interfere with sexual function range from minor conditions, such as a rigid hymen, which may require a small surgical incision under anaesthesia to allow intercourse, to more complex abnormalities requiring major surgical intervention.

A woman with a rigid hymen at least has an opening that allows menstrual flow. In contrast, an imperforate hymen causes severe cyclical lower abdominal pain due to retained menstrual blood. On examination, the hymen appears as a tense, bluish bulge, and a cruciate incision relieves the obstruction, restores normal menstruation, and allows for future sexual activity.

Other conditions, such as a uterine septum, can cause reproductive difficulties but are amenable to treatment. However, some anomalies remain difficult or impossible to correct. These include a bicornuate uterus—a double uterus with one cervix, two uteri with two cervices, or absence of the cervix or uterus. Uterine transplants are now being attempted at select centres. These pose reproductive difficulties, though intercourse is possible. On the other hand, an absent vagina can be constructed surgically, while a vaginal septum, transverse, or longitudinal can be excised to improve sexual function.

Suffice it to say that, though rare, abnormalities of the genital tract must be considered and addressed whenever a woman presents with coital difficulties.

Part V

When Pleasure Has Consequences

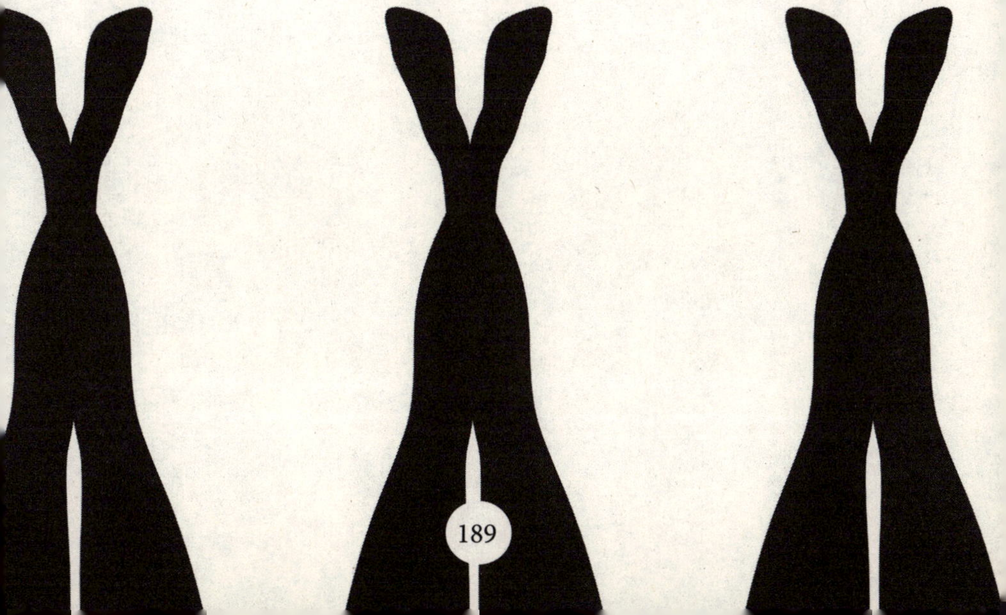

24

A Burning Issue

Rhea had an arranged marriage with the suave, gallant Saurabh and had fallen in love with him during their engagement. Being a virgin, she looked forward to their honeymoon in the Maldives, where they would consummate the marriage. Coyly, she sat in their cottage in the midst of a pristine blue sea, which suddenly exploded into a splash of colours as it reflected the setting sun. Even as the golden globe sank into the bosom of the sea, her husband sank on to hers. Her sexuality was a bud that he opened gently, petal by petal, and in the process was rewarded by the sweet nectar she exuded. Her breath caught as he breached her hymen and entered her but, despite the pain, she allowed him to continue till he collapsed on her in a gratified heap.

There were no fireworks as she had expected. It usually never is the first time around for a woman, but she could not help feeling a bit disappointed. However, as the days passed, her husband's expertise (whether gleaned from books or from previous experiences, she dared not ask) and her eagerness to learn soon introduced her to the pleasures of sex and the ecstasy of an orgasm. In fact, she could not have enough of it. They barely explored the beauty of the locale, so engrossed were they in exploring the beauty of their bodies, but that was what a honeymoon was all about.

All too soon, the ecstasy turned to agony. One morning, Saurabh needed to use the washroom urgently and Rhea was taking her own sweet time. He was about to bang on the door in exasperation when he heard sobs emanating from within. Alarmed, he entered to learn that she was experiencing intense burning as one acidic drop of urine fell after the other. Each time she got up, she felt the urge to pee again but dared not let go on account of the excruciating pain. He wiped her tears, held her to his chest, and offered her a glass of water, which she refused lest it increase her desire for urination. The next time she went to the toilet, she was horrified to see that she was passing blood instead of urine. They rang up their family doctor, who advised an alkaliser, but it offered scant relief. Soon her symptoms became so unbearable that they had to cut short their honeymoon and return home.

A visit to the gynaecologist revealed that she was suffering from 'Honeymoon Cystitis'. Cystitis is the medical term for inflammation of the bladder, which is usually caused by bacterial infection. It commonly follows sexual activity in women, the risk increasing with the frequency of sex. As the frequency is maximum during the honeymoon period, UTIs occurring at this time is also called 'honeymoon cystitis'.

The female anatomy has a major role to play in the frequency of UTI in women. Unlike the male, her urethra (the tube that connects the bladder to the outside) is short, and its meatus (opening) is in close proximity to the vagina. It is also closer to the anus as compared to males. As a result, bacteria have to travel a very short distance to reach the bladder. Sexual intercourse can push bacteria into the urethra, from where they ascend to the bladder and infect it. Another common factor is the use of a jet while washing after defecation. Water sprayed from back to front pushes bacteria present in the stools forward to infect the urinary tract. A woman can suffer from a UTI at any time in her life, but pregnancy, diabetes, and stones are predisposing factors. Its frequency increases again after menopause because the vagina becomes thin and dry. This is due to decreased levels of female hormones, which also affect the base of the bladder.

Symptoms, as we have seen above, include a persistent urge to urinate, frequent passage of small amounts of urine, burning during urination, blood in the urine, and low-grade fever. At times, the kidneys get infected (pyelonephritis), in which case there is high fever with chills, nausea, vomiting, and pain in the flanks. This is a serious condition that may need hospitalisation and IV antibiotics.

Investigations

Routine urine examination will reveal large quantities of pus cells, red blood cells, and bacteria. Urine culture and sensitivity will give information about the infective organism (the commonest being *E. coli*) and the antibiotic to which it is sensitive. At times, a KUB (ultrasound of the kidneys and urinary bladder) is done to look for stones, growths, and dilatation of the urinary tract. Cystoscopy is done when a bladder stone or growth is suspected.

Treatment

Contrary to what people think, one must increase the intake of oral fluids to dilute the urine and flush out bacteria; cranberry juice helps. Urinary alkalisers neutralise the acidity of urine and decrease the burning sensation; urinary analgesics offer relief from pain, while antibiotics get rid of the bacteria. A full course should be taken to prevent the development of resistance. In those who have infrequent intercourse but are prone to UTI after sex, a single antibiotic pill immediately afterwards prevents sex-related cystitis. Pregnancy limits our choice of antibiotics, as only those safe for the growing foetus can be prescribed. Postmenopausal women are also prescribed vaginal oestrogen creams because the posterior wall of the bladder is in close proximity to the anterior vaginal wall and responds to local replacement of female hormones. Recurrent or chronic UTI requires prolonged antibiotic therapy.

Asymptomatic Bacteriuria

Sometimes, bacteria are found in the urine sample but cause no symptoms. There is no need for antibiotics in these women, with one exception—pregnancy, when antibiotics are given even if there are no symptoms, to decrease the incidence of miscarriage, low birth-weight babies, and preterm births associated with it.

Pregnancy increases the incidence of asymptomatic bacilluria due to hormone-associated changes in the bladder, such as reduced bladder tone that leads to urinary stasis. This allows bacteria to grow and ascend to the kidneys, leading to pyelonephritis, which occurs in 30–45 per cent of women with untreated asymptomatic bacilluria, resulting in the above-mentioned pregnancy complications.

Prevention

Drink plenty of water (cranberry juice may reduce the risk of recurrent bladder infections); avoid caffeinated drinks. Do not hold urine for prolonged periods, as this gives bacteria time to grow. Pass urine immediately after sex. Drinking water after intercourse increases the amount of urine, which flushes out bacteria. Try positions like woman on top when the urethral opening is not subjected to friction. Use vaginal lubricant in case of dryness; oestrogen creams help in postmenopausal women. Wipe or wash the genital area from front to back after a bowel movement to prevent bacteria in the anal region from being carried forward to the vagina and urethra. Take showers instead of tub baths. Wash the local area with mild soap or plain water to prevent irritation of the delicate skin in this region. Avoid deodorant sprays or feminine hygiene products in the local area, as they may irritate the urethra and bladder.

Vaginal Discharge and STIs

Women, especially those who have newly stepped into adulthood, are very concerned about vaginal discharge. It could be physiological or pathological. Physiological discharge is not malodorous. It varies in consistency and quantity during different phases of the menstrual cycle. It tends to be thick and white in the pre- and postmenstrual phase, and thin and transparent mid-cycle around the time of ovulation, to make the birth canal accessible to sperm for fertilisation. At the time of sexual excitement, Bartholin's glands, situated on either side of the vaginal opening, secrete a thin, slimy discharge for lubrication.

Unhealthy vaginal discharge in sexually active women could be a sign of a sexually transmitted infection (STI). Any discharge that is malodorous, greenish, or yellowish in colour, and/or associated with itching or burning is due to infection and needs treatment. Eradication of the infection should be complete and thorough so that the condition does not become chronic or recurrent. It is important to simultaneously treat the woman's sexual partner(s) to prevent reinfection.

Young girls with immature genital tracts who indulge in sexual activity, as well as pregnant and postmenopausal women, are more prone to vaginal infections.

Causes

These include poor personal hygiene. Tight undergarments or underwear made of synthetic material like nylon, douches, and allergic or chemical reactions to deodorants and soaps can lead to vulvovaginitis. Hormonal disturbances, oral contraceptives, intrauterine contraceptive devices, and worm infestation—chiefly pinworms—are other causes. An intrauterine contraceptive device or cervical erosion, characterised by redness of the cervix (which should be pink like the vagina), increases discharge, which becomes unhealthy and foul-smelling if secondary infection occurs. Foreign bodies such as diaphragms, condoms, tampons, or objects inserted in the vagina during masturbation could also be the reason. Antibiotics taken for any reason destroy good vaginal bacteria, allowing harmful bacteria to infect. Last but not least are STIs (sexually transmitted infections).

STIs know no barriers of age, socio-economic status, or ethnicity, for any sexually active woman can get infected. They spread through oral, genital, or anal sex. The commonest STIs are:

Candida

This is a fungal infection of the lower genital area that causes intense itching and thick, curdy white discharge. The local area is red and swollen, and there is burning during urination. While a large proportion of people infected with Candida remain symptom-free, they can act as carriers and infect their sex partners. Diabetes, pregnancy, and contraceptive pills make a woman more susceptible to fungal infection. The recurrence rate is high, so both partners should be treated to bring about a complete cure.

Trichomoniasis

This is characterised by the flow of a copious, foul-smelling, frothy greenish-yellow discharge. It is accompanied by soreness of the external genitalia and pain during urination and intercourse.

Bacterial Vaginosis

There is a thin, skimmed-milk-like discharge with a fishy odour. There are no signs of inflammation, such as soreness or swelling.

Chlamydia

This is the commonest sexually transmitted disease. Though it can permanently damage the upper genital system, leading to infertility and chronic pelvic pain, it remains asymptomatic in as many as 70 per cent of cases. Those who have symptoms present with yellowish-green vaginal discharge. They may have urinary symptoms such as burning and pus discharge, though the urine culture report is usually sterile. There may be inflammation of the rectum and 'pink eye'—red-rimmed eyes due to inflammation of the conjunctiva. It can cause pelvic inflammatory disease (PID), characterised by backache, lower abdominal pain, and painful intercourse, which wrecks a person's sex life.

If the acute infection is not treated, it becomes chronic. PID can lead to blocked tubes, infertility, ectopic pregnancy, and chronic pelvic pain. If a woman does conceive, it can lead to preterm delivery and infect the newborn. As the clinical signs and symptoms are rare and the long-term sequelae are high, the condition has to be actively looked for and treated vigorously.

Gonorrhoea

This STD has long-term effects similar to chlamydia but manifests early in the form of unhealthy vaginal discharge and pain while passing urine, though at times this, too, may be asymptomatic. Anal sex results in rectal pain, while oral sex can cause a sore throat. The disease, however, can be cured completely by appropriate antibiotics. If left untreated, it may cause PID. The eyes of the foetus can be damaged during vaginal delivery in a patient with gonorrhoea, leading to blindness.

Other STIs cause local lesions instead of vaginal discharge. These include:

Syphilis

After an incubation period of about three weeks, a single hard, painless swelling appears in the genital region. Those indulging in extragenital sex may have lesions on the lips, mouth, nipples, and anus. The 'chancre', as the lesion is called, gradually erodes and ulcerates. The ulcer is painless, punched out, with clean, raised borders. As it may develop deep in the vagina and is painless, the woman may be unaware that she has syphilis. This leads to a delay in treatment and spread of the disease to her sex partners. The chancre heals of its own accord within a few weeks. If untreated, syphilis progresses to the secondary stage, characterised by a symmetrical bilateral skin rash, particularly on the palms and soles.

Condyloma—polypoid growths—may appear in warm, moist areas like the perineum, the area between the genitals, and the anus. These lesions are highly infective. After a latent period (when the disease is not infective), 30 per cent of patients progress to the tertiary stage, which may involve the vascular and neurological systems. A mother can infect her unborn child at any stage. The chances of stillbirths and neonatal deaths (death within seven days of birth) are very high. It is for this reason that all pregnant women are tested for syphilis and treated if found to be positive. At times, a live baby is born with signs of congenital syphilis.

Penicillin is the drug of choice in all stages of syphilis, though other drugs are given to those sensitive to penicillin. Sexual activity can be resumed seven to ten days after completion of therapy or once the lesions have completely healed.

Genital Herpes

This is a viral infection that occurs after genital or oro-genital sexual contact with an infected partner. The chances of infection are as high as 75 per cent. The incubation period is two to ten days. There may be fever and general malaise. Primary infection presents as painful, fluid-filled blisters on the external genitalia, accompanied by dysuria (pain while passing urine). After some time, the lesions burst, leaving behind shallow, painful ulcers that crust and heal in one to two weeks without leaving any scars. However, it may take two to four weeks to recover from the first outbreak.

Recurrent infection can occur within a period of one to three months, though recovery is faster, within three to seven days. It is usually triggered by mental stress, menstrual distress, intercourse, and insomnia. Before secondary lesions appear, there is tingling or itching in the local area. Genital herpes responds very well to antiviral drugs. Special care has to be taken in a pregnant woman, as the infection is likely to spread to the newborn. If active lesions are present at the time of birth, a caesarean section is the preferred mode of delivery.

Human Papillomavirus (HPV)

Human papillomavirus occurs predominantly in the age group of fifteen to thirty years. The latent period is three months or even longer. There are over one hundred strains of the HPV virus, some of which lead to the formation of genital warts, while others lead to genital cancer. This is one STI that cannot be prevented by the use of condoms, as it spreads by skin-to-skin contact. The recurrence rate is high, either due to an untreated partner or the presence of latent virus beneath normal-looking skin.

Clinically, it presents as multiple fleshy warts growing over the external genitalia and extending up to the perineum and anus. Treatment consists of local application of toxic drugs such as podophyllin at weekly intervals. If unsuccessful or if the woman is pregnant, cryotherapy or laser ablation can be tried, but the warts tend to recur.

Certain strains of HPV lead to cancer of the cervix (the mouth of the uterus). It is found to be the cause in as many as 85 per cent of cases of cervical cancer. A Pap smear is the testing of cervical fluid for cancer or precancerous conditions. To diagnose the presence of carcinogenic strains of HPV, the same sample can also be tested for the virus. If positive, do not panic, for the good news is that the virus takes about ten years to progress into cancer. In the meantime, though there is no cure, most healthy people get rid of it on their own, as seen by a negative HPV report when tested at six-monthly intervals.

Persistent HPV infection must be actively looked for and followed up. The protocol in India, and in most other countries, is as follows: Pap smear or liquid-based cytology (LBC), a better version of Pap smear, should be repeated every three years, starting at the age of twenty-one. After thirty, till sixty-five, it should be combined with HPV testing and repeated every five years if negative. Those who do not test for HPV (the reasons could be non-availability of the test or the cost) can continue with a Pap smear or LBC every three years. This will diagnose precancerous conditions or early cancer, which is 100 per cent treatable. A suspicious Pap smear followed by colposcopy and cervical biopsy can confirm the diagnosis and treat it simultaneously.

Nowadays, a vaccine is available against the virus. It can be given to every woman between the ages of nine and forty-five, in two to three doses (depending on age), at intervals prescribed by the company that manufactures it. Vaccination of both boys and girls, along with regular Pap smears, can help eradicate cervical cancer, which is one of the most common cancers in India.

Other STIs have no symptoms most of the time but can cause havoc. These include:

HIV and AIDS

This deserves an entire chapter and has been given that honour.

Hepatitis B Virus (HBV)

This infection is caused by a virus that is one hundred times more infectious than AIDS and kills more people in a day than AIDS kills in a year. Like AIDS, it is a major cause of death in the prime of life; however, unlike HIV, there is an effective vaccine available for the prevention of HBV. Moreover, there is no stigma attached to the disease. One in twenty Indians is a carrier, making India the second-largest carrier pool in the world. It is alarming that most carriers are unaware that they are HBV carriers. Nearly 30 per cent of these patients ultimately die of complications such as cirrhosis and liver cancer.

A carrier should avoid sharing personal items that may have blood on them, such as razors, toothbrushes, and nail cutters, and should get the rest of the family immunised against the disease. He or she should avoid drugs that can damage the liver, get liver function tests done on a regular basis, and go for follow-up visits throughout life.

The highest concentration of this virus is found in blood, followed by semen, vaginal secretions, and wound exudates. Sexual transmission accounts for most adult hepatitis B virus (HBV) infections. Approximately 25 per cent of those in regular sexual contact with an infected individual will themselves become infected. In turn, 10–20 per cent of infected pregnant women will transmit the infection to their babies. This can be prevented by giving appropriate vaccination at birth. All pregnant women are tested for HBV infection.

The incubation period is between six weeks and six months. Only half of the patients with acute HBV infection are symptomatic and present with loss of appetite, nausea, vomiting, fever, abdominal pain, and jaundice. Treatment is supportive, as there is no cure. In the acute phase, transmission to the baby is up to 10 per cent in the first trimester and as high as 80–90 per cent in the third trimester.

Prevention of STIs

Use plain water or mild soap in the genital region instead of scented soaps, detergents, feminine hygiene products, or douching. Take a shower instead of soaking in a bathtub and avoid sitting in wet clothes, such as bathing suits for prolonged periods. Avoid tight clothes, synthetic underwear, and talc in the genital region, as these block the openings of sweat glands. Trim pubic hair instead of shaving or waxing. Clean the genital area from front to back so that infection does not spread from the anal region to the genital area.

Sexually active women should practise safe sex, avoid multiple sex partners, and encourage the use of a condom even in a monogamous relationship, as the partner may or may not be monogamous. A new sexual partner should not be encouraged during pregnancy. Any foul-smelling or yellowish discharge, itching, burning, sores, or warts in the genital area should be reported.

The havoc wrought by STIs can make a woman a sexual or reproductive cripple for life. This manifests as chronic pelvic pain, pain during intercourse, menstrual irregularities, infertility, and general debility. Hence, it is imperative that medical advice is sought as soon as anything untoward is noticed. Specific treatment should be started at the right time, in the right dose, and for the appropriate duration. It is mandatory that both sexual partners be treated, even if the male partner has no complaints, as he could be a carrier. This will prevent reinfection.

25

Living with HIV

It was daunting to learn that there are people in the world who desperately want to end their lives but do not have the courage to do so. I was of the opinion that suicide was an act o cowardice. The question smote me afresh when a lower-middle-class woman came to my clinic one afternoon. She wanted me to give her poison to end her life. I scolded her roundly, well-acquainted with high-strung females who brought their domestic squabbles to my office. If they wanted to scare their husbands with the pretence of suicide, there were other means. Soon, the curiosity of a writer overcame the annoyance of a doctor, and I asked, 'Why do you want to die?'

'That I can't tell you. Just give me the poison.' As if I were a minion at her beck and call.

I stared at her. She was a presentable-looking young woman who seemed healthy enough.

'Are you pregnant?' I asked, thinking that if it was an illegitimate pregnancy worrying her, she could kill the baby, not herself.

'No, that is . . . not now. I got it aborted.'

'Why?'

'I already have three children.'

'And you want to leave them in the lurch.'

'Their father will look after them.'

'I am asking for the last time, why do you want to die?'

'I cannot tell you,' she repeated stubbornly.

'Then go away.'

She neither moved nor said anything. Just then, a thought struck me like lightning.

'Are you HIV positive?' I asked. It was the latest scourge those many years ago, and a much-dreaded one.

'Something along those lines.'

'How did you come to know?'

'By a blood test.'

'And why did you get your blood tested?'

'They tested it before performing the abortion.'

'Get your husband tested, too. He must have given the infection to you,' I said, pitying the poor woman.

'He is not that sort.' Indeed! Could a woman be so naïve?

'How can you be so sure?' I asked.

'I made the mistake myself.'

'What?'

'I committed a wrong.'

'With whom?'

'With my husband's friend. He seduced me, and we had sex off and on. Later, I learnt that he had relations with other women, too.'

It took me a while to digest this. If I had crossed this woman on the street, I would never have thought that this *gharelu*, Sati Savitri prototype of ideal Indian womanhood could be anything, but a docile wife devoted to her Pati Parmeshwar.

'How long have you known about the disease?'

'About a month.'

'And the baby? Who was the father?'

'I was not sure . . .'

'What about that man?'

'He left me when he learnt about the pregnancy.'

'And your husband? Does he know?'

'Yes. The doctor said that he should get tested, too; he refused.'

'What if he has contracted the infection from you? Your children will be orphaned.'

'My fifteen-year-old daughter will look after her two brothers.'

'Listen, you are merely HIV positive. It takes up to eight to ten years for it to develop into full-fledged AIDS. That is the time to contemplate suicide, not now. You could get your children settled in the meantime.'

'I have no will to live. My sins are beyond redemption.'

'Living in such a mental state is punishment enough,' I said sanctimoniously.

'Please give me the poison.'

The tears that had welled up all this time turned into heart-wrenching sobs.

'I do not keep poison on my premises,' I said gently.

'Please . . .' she begged.

'It is not so dreadful as you think. Medicines prolong the AIDS-free interval in an HIV-positive patient. With time, you will learn to live with it,' I said gently.

'I don't want to live . . . with or without the disease. I cannot stand being beaten mercilessly day after day and raped brutally night after night by a raving mad husband.'

'What?! But why does he want to sleep with you despite—'

'Men will be men. How can I stop him?' she interjected.

I was shocked. In all probability, he was HIV positive, too. What more could he lose when all was lost already? This was his revenge and, in a perverted sort of way, his rejection.

'But, but . . .' I sputtered.

'I live in dread of the day when my daughter learns the truth,' she sobbed.

Nothing could assuage her shame, guilt, pain, and regret. The disease had mauled her psyche much before it would ravage her flesh, and she writhed in agony. Whichever way I looked at it, she was doomed.

I reflected upon the article—complete with impersonal data—that I had written in a dispassionate way about AIDS for a magazine. To be confronted in flesh and blood by just one of those who was a mere statistic in the report unnerved me, a seasoned practitioner accustomed to the vagaries of life and the consistency of death. That she carried the seed of a shameful death in her healthy-looking body was difficult to contemplate. Never was a person more needed by life than this young mother, the pivot around which her growing family revolved, yet she was being chased by the demons of despair down a one-way street to her doom. Mutely, I watched the complete disintegration of a human being.

'Please . . .' she begged one last time.

'I cannot,' I said, averting my gaze from her haunted eyes.

Defeated, she got up to go. As I watched her leave with drooping shoulders and dragging steps, her little son running after her, I wondered if I would have done her a service by letting her have her way. Suddenly, an idea struck me. My next posting would, perhaps, be in the AIDS ward.

Five years later . . .

The morning rush over, Sumitra served piping hot tea, prepared exactly the way I liked it, and sat on the low stool beside me, sipping hers as we enjoyed our brief respite from work. Despite our difference in class, we had become friends. The lady once desperate to end her life had found her calling. I got her a job as a GDA (general duty attendant) in the AIDS wards of our hospital, where I was unit in-charge. It was a job she did diligently and with compassion, one that most others were reluctant to do. She had nothing to lose and everything to gain.

With her dignity restored and a steady source of income, she shifted out of her abusive husband's home with her children. Her daughter was as hardworking as she was. After school, she did the housework and helped her two younger brothers with their homework. She had won a scholarship and would soon join college. All was well with Sumitra's world again. She could now live in peace and, when the time came, die in peace. As of now, her antiretroviral medicines were doing their job; she had not progressed to AIDS and, God willing, would live long enough to see her family settled.

HIV and AIDS

HIV (human immunodeficiency virus) is a virus that attacks the body's immune system. If left untreated, it can lead to AIDS (acquired immunodeficiency syndrome), the scourge of modern times. This deficiency in the immune system allows opportunistic infections to invade the body and eventually kill it. A disease of young, sexually active people, it had spread in epidemic proportions a few decades ago. Though it remains a global epidemic, HIV has been somewhat contained over the years. Unlike the early eighties, when it was first discovered, it has become a chronic disease with a drastic decrease in death rates since its peak in 1995. This is because, though there is still no cure, progression to AIDS can be stalled with drugs.

As there are no visible signs in the initial stage—it takes years for the disease to progress into its full-fledged lethal form—the infected person can spread the disease even though he or she appears healthy. All sexually active people are at risk, but the most vulnerable are teenagers and pregnant women. Adolescence represents a time of hormonal surge, which prompts risk-taking behaviour in the form of sexual experimentation with multiple partners and drug abuse. Added to this is total ignorance about the hazards of unprotected sex and sharing of needles among drug abusers, which is an open invitation to HIV. Homosexuality and promiscuity are additional factors; in fact, the disease was first discovered in homosexual males.

Not all young men and women are sex-crazed drug addicts, but what if a virgin gets married to a normal-looking person who is HIV positive? She will contract the disease through no fault of hers, as will her offspring, for a pregnant HIV-positive woman has a 20–30 per cent chance of transferring the disease to her unborn child. Instead of matching horoscopes before marriage, matching the couple's HIV status would be far more beneficial.

What Is AIDS?

AIDS is an acronym for Acquired Immunodeficiency Syndrome, caused by a retrovirus called the human immunodeficiency virus (HIV). This selectively infects and destroys a certain type of white blood cells, the CD4 cells, which are responsible for the immunological response of the body. A decrease in the CD4 cell count leads to failure of the body's defence mechanism, resulting in an onslaught of opportunistic infections, as the body is unable to resist organisms that invade the weakened system. The patient eventually succumbs to serious secondary infections.

HIV is acquired through homosexual or heterosexual contact or contact with body fluids of an infected individual—blood and blood products, tears, saliva, and breast milk; by sharing needles with an infected person, as seen among drug addicts; and through transfusion of infected blood or blood products. Infected mothers can transmit the infection to their offspring during pregnancy, delivery, or breastfeeding. Health workers can accidentally be inoculated with the virus through needle-prick injuries or contact with body fluids on mucosa or broken skin. People with other STIs have a greater chance of acquiring the disease than the general population.

Surprisingly, the virus is so delicate that even soap and water or household bleach can destroy it.

HIV does not spread through casual contact, sharing food, utensils, clothing, or toilet seats; shaking hands; dry kissing or hugging; insect bites; or masturbation. Nor does it spread by living or working with an HIV-positive person. Massages and sexual stimulation will not spread the disease, provided care is taken to prevent contact of body fluids or blood with broken skin or mucosa.

Course of the Disease

There are three stages of HIV infection. Symptoms vary in type and severity from person to person, with some experiencing no symptoms in the first two stages.

Stage 1

One to four weeks after exposure, following initial infection, flu-like symptoms may occur, though not everyone experiences them. Despite being infected and capable of spreading the disease, the person tests negative for HIV during this 'window period'. Hence, the importance of prevention through the use of condoms; drug abusers should not share needles. Seroconversion (testing positive for HIV) can take anywhere from four weeks to six months.

Stage 2

Many people start to feel better. Though HIV positive, they remain asymptomatic for eight to ten years or even longer but can still spread the disease.

Stage 3

The immune system breaks down and can no longer fight off serious infections, which eventually kill the patient. Symptoms include weight loss, chronic diarrhoea, night sweats, fever, persistent cough, and mouth and skin problems. Once opportunistic infections take over, a person becomes a full-blown case of AIDS. Tuberculosis has returned in a big way on account of the lowered resistance of the body due to AIDS. Herpes, oral thrush (a furry white growth in the mouth and food pipe due to the fungus *Candida*), Kaposi's sarcoma (a form of skin cancer), and a rare variety of intractable pneumonia are some of the infections that invade a body weakened by the virus.

Treatment

Though there is no cure, treatment is aimed at controlling the disease, managing secondary infections, and rebuilding the body's defence mechanism. Antiretroviral drugs (ART) are the mainstay of treatment and, thankfully, can be given to pregnant women as well. They act by preventing replication of the virus, which in turn helps keep the person's immune system strong. This delays the onset of AIDS by several years. However, ART has to be taken every day for the rest of the person's life. A lot depends upon the age and prior health status of the individual, the viral load, and the number of CD4 cells in the body. The earlier the disease is diagnosed, the earlier treatment is initiated, and the stricter the adherence to therapy, the better the prognosis. People on ART with no detectable level of virus in their blood will not spread the virus to their sexual partners.

The stigma and discrimination associated with HIV/AIDS lead to feelings of shame and lack of self-worth, which compromise mental health. Therefore, addressing a patient's mental health is as important as managing physical issues. A multifaceted approach will improve quality of life, and besides adding years to life, it will add life to years.

Rock Hudson and Freddie Mercury, the famous actor and singer, were among those who died of AIDS—beautiful, talented men who, on account of the associated shame, kept their homosexuality and affliction under wraps until just before death. Medicine has come a long way since then. Antiretroviral therapy delays the progression of HIV to AIDS, which is the eventual killer. An HIV-positive individual can now lead a healthy, productive life for many years.

26

Unwanted Pregnancies: Abortions

Besides STIs, unwanted pregnancies are the most important by-product of unprotected sex, though they are perceived as easier to get rid of. Any woman above the age of eighteen, whether married or unmarried, with or without the knowledge or consent of her partner or husband, can legally undergo a medical termination of pregnancy (MTP), often by taking a few pills. The social and emotional implications, however, are an entirely different matter.

Surprisingly, the predominant emotion I see in most cases is relief rather than guilt, which is what I might have expected. Social repercussions can range from separation to divorce if a woman chooses to terminate a pregnancy that her husband or in-laws want her to continue, though the opposite can also be true. A woman may opt for an abortion expressly because she wants to opt out of the marriage, and a child would be an encumbrance. At times, pregnant women are forced to abort a female foetus even when they wish to continue the pregnancy. More commonly, however, women seek abortions for less pressing reasons—career concerns, an unplanned pregnancy soon after marriage or after the birth of a first child, or the desire to 'get to know each other better', as most marriages in India are still arranged.

Pre-marital or pre-conception counselling for contraception is rarely sought. As a result, newlyweds, recently introduced to the pleasures of sex, are reluctant to be burdened by an offspring conceived in the process. I try to ask such couples to rethink their decision before taking this irreversible step by apprising them of possible consequences, including infertility. Some are convinced; others are not.

I recall a colleague with whom I had lost contact after he moved to another area. On seeing his daughter's photograph in the newspaper—she was a junior-level national tennis champion—I called to congratulate him.

'*Aap ki beti ki photo newspaper mein dekh kar bahut khushi hui* [I was very pleased to see your daughter's photograph in the newspaper].'

'*Hamari beti kahan? Yeh toh aap ki beti hai* [Not our daughter. She is your daughter].'

Agreed! I had delivered her, but that made me her godmother at best, not her mother. When I responded with an unconvincing 'Of course,' he reminded me that they had come to me for an abortion because the child had been conceived just six months after the birth of their elder daughter. Being a radiologist, he knew the foetus was female. I had convinced them to continue with the pregnancy, and this very girl had made them proud. This reminded me of a true story I read years ago in *Reader's Digest*. While delivering a breech (bottom-first) baby girl, the doctor noticed that one leg was shorter than the other. Wanting to spare the child a life of misery, he briefly contemplated delaying the delivery of the after-coming head so that the baby would asphyxiate. Thankfully, his conscience prevailed. The girl survived and went on to become a famous musician.

Complications

While some women undergo multiple abortions without apparent complications, I have seen others suffer devastating consequences even after their very first procedure. Immediate complications include perforation of the uterus, with or without injury to internal organs such as the bladder or intestines; incomplete abortion; continuation of pregnancy; and acute pelvic infection. Infection may progress to chronic pelvic inflammatory disease (PID), manifesting as chronic pelvic pain, pain during menstruation or intercourse, menstrual irregularities, blocked fallopian tubes, and infertility.

A woman may develop uterine synechiae, where the inner walls of the uterus adhere to each other, resulting in scanty periods or amenorrhoea. She may also develop an ectopic pregnancy, in which the foetus implants outside the uterus, most commonly in the fallopian tube. If not diagnosed and managed in time, the tube with the ectopic pregnancy can rupture, leading to profuse internal bleeding that could be fatal.

It is important that every patient seeking an MTP be made aware of these risks. Sadly, most women would rather terminate a pregnancy than prevent one. This is because MTP is perceived as a relatively safe procedure when done early, in the right setup, by the right personnel. All that is required is to tick 'failure of contraception' as the reason on the MTP form. Nowadays, women also have the option of abortion pills, which ideally should be taken under medical supervision but are often sold over the counter by unscrupulous chemists. To avoid the expense of a doctor's consultation and the ultrasound that is usually advised, many women self-medicate. This is being penny-wise and pound-foolish, as I have seen near-fatal consequences.

An ultrasound determines the location and size of the pregnancy and detects twins or coexisting fibroids. In the rare instance of an ectopic pregnancy, taking abortion pills can be catastrophic. Medical abortion is not always complete; retained products of conception (RPOC) may require surgical removal, and torrential bleeding can occur. It is therefore wise to remain in touch with a doctor while undergoing a pill-induced abortion so that help is immediately available if needed.

Moreover, these pills are effective only up to a certain gestational age. Women who take them for more advanced pregnancies often pay a heavy price for poor judgement.

The larger the pregnancy, the more difficult it is to terminate. For years, twenty weeks was the upper legal limit for abortion; this has recently been increased to twenty-four weeks in select cases, such as severe foetal malformations. Termination at this stage requires induction of labour, and on occasion, the foetus may be born alive.

After years of practice, very little shocks me anymore. Not the girl raped by her father, not the domestic worker impregnated by her employer, not the fifteen-year-old with an eighteen-week pregnancy whose only complaint was that her jeans had become tight, not the impoverished family of eight who, for monetary compensation, offered their eldest daughter to a tea-stall owner and subjected her to repeated abortions. I once caught a ward boy attempting to photograph the exposed genitals of a girl under anaesthesia, and a hospital *ayah* trying to extort money from an unmarried woman who had come for a mid-trimester abortion. I put an end to both.

With age, my cynicism grew, but I could not stomach the thought of unscrupulous health professionals exploiting hapless unmarried girls. My blood still boils when I think of one such incident. I was called to manage a 'complication' at a small nursing home in a colony. Accustomed to helping colleagues in distress, I went, unaware of the vile intent brewing there.

I was unaware of their history of sexually assaulting sedated, unmarried girls. This particular patient was insisting that only a female doctor perform her abortion. Their plan was for me to stay until she was deeply sedated, step out while they raped her, and then return to perform the MTP. Sick to my stomach, I turned around and walked out. I would have reported them to the police, but the girl's reputation was at stake, and the police were no better at 'handling' such cases. Had I possessed a gun at that moment, I might have used it.

In another case, surgeons struggled to remove a massive stone from a young girl's urinary bladder. Oddly, it extended beyond the posterior bladder wall into the vagina. As a gynaecologist, I was called in. To our horror, we discovered that the stone had formed around a pen cap. The girl had tried to induce an abortion by inserting a pen into her vagina. Instead of entering the uterus, it perforated the vaginal wall and entered the bladder. When she attempted to pull it out, the cap remained inside. Terrified, she told no one.

Then there was a baby who survived our attempts to terminate it. When the woman failed to menstruate a month after the procedure, an ultrasound revealed a live, growing foetus. As the family still did not want the child, I was asked to help, this time under ultrasound guidance. To our astonishment, while our instrument entered the uterine cavity on one side, the foetus appeared to be on the other. No matter how hard we tried, we could not reach it.

The woman had a rare uterine anomaly—an accessory horn communicating with the main uterine cavity through a tiny opening. The pregnancy was safely nestled there. The baby survived our repeated attempts and was eventually delivered by caesarean section. I can only hope that fate had something extraordinary in store for the child.

Hired Assassins

Though my mother became a doctor vicariously through me, she soon began dictating terms that I found impossible to follow. The Medical Termination of Pregnancy (MTP) Act had just been passed, and she wanted me to promise her that I would not 'take' lives. I was a mere house surgeon then, expected to do what was asked of me and not question why.

Yet I could not stop wondering: How could something that was a sin in the eyes of God receive legal sanction? My conscience remained at loggerheads with the call of duty until a fateful night in the emergency room. A young girl was wheeled in, her relatives screaming that a 'snake' was slithering out of her private parts. The hapless teenager lay on the stretcher in shock (this is medical shock when the skin is cold and clammy, the pulse is fast, and BP is low, with or without loss of consciousness). When I lifted the sheet, I froze in horror: A two-foot-long loop of intestines was protruding from her vagina.

While attempting to abort an illegitimate pregnancy, an untrained 'nurse' had pierced the uterus with a steel instrument, entered the abdominal cavity, and pulled out whatever her unrelenting grip could grasp—a long, glistening structure she mistook for a snake. Needless to say, we lost the girl. Perhaps she was better off dead than alive in the given circumstances, but after witnessing such a horrific end to a promising young life, I understood why the MTP Act had been passed. It saved women who would otherwise have succumbed to infection, bleeding, or organ injury following clandestine abortions performed at seedy centres by untrained *dais*.

Yet this understanding did not erase the pang I felt each time I had to destroy an unsuspecting little one, snug within the supposed safety of its mother's womb. Little did it know that the very parents who had given it life were now conspiring with the doctor to get rid of it.

The question haunted me: Who was the sinner—the mother, the father, the doctor, or all three? This moral conundrum troubled me deeply until I sternly told myself to stop overthinking. A hired assassin who develops a soft spot for his victim will never be able to do justice to his profession.

Today, we have pills to abort pregnancies at an early stage, and the doctor's role is often limited to guidance and, at times, removal of retained products of conception. Alternatively, the pregnancy is sucked out through a cannula attached to a suction tube and lands in a glass bottle as a small blob of blood mixed with barely visible mincemeat of what could have been a promising life. As this does not remotely resemble a human being, it becomes easier to pretend that it is not one.

Abortions are legal up to twenty weeks (twenty-four weeks in special cases where severe malformations are detected late). Termination at this stage causes immense suffering to the woman, who must endure painful uterine contractions to expel the foetus, which sometimes emerges alive, leaving her physically and emotionally depleted.

What troubled me most then, and troubles me even now after years of practice, are MTPs performed between eleven and thirteen weeks of pregnancy, when body parts begin to form. In fact, the gutted feeling these procedures left me with prompted the beginning of my writing career . . . with a bang!

I wrote an article titled *The Silent Cry* after reading about an ultrasound image (a rarity in those days) captured during an abortion. It showed the foetus recoiling in terror, backing away, and opening its mouth in a silent scream. The article was published in *Woman's Era* and created a furore. A debate ensued, and the magazine was flooded with letters. The best three arguments for and against MTP were rewarded. Though I no longer have the original article, what follows is another piece written along similar lines.

A satisfied customer referred this couple to me. They wanted to get rid of someone close, and I was a professional with considerable experience in the art of elimination. What did I care, as long as they paid my fee upfront? Without bargaining, they placed the money on the table.

'His crime?' I asked, not particularly interested—though the answer intrigued me.

'His very existence.' That he dared to live when they did not want him to was provocation enough. Whatever the reason, it did not concern me. My job was to perform efficiently and satisfy my client.

I was handed a photograph—a black-and-white one (an ultrasound)—that confirmed his location and physical attributes, including age and size. After planning the modus operandi down to the minutest detail, we fixed a date and time. This one seemed inordinately fond of water; he spent most of his time in the bathtub. I decided to finish him off there.

As the door was secured by a heavy latch, it needed tampering in advance. In the early days, I would wedge a piece of special wood—a dried seaweed—at this strategic point. It absorbed moisture and swelled overnight, loosening the portal and making my job easier. These days, I have better tools at my disposal that work faster and require less effort.

Having set the scene, I donned the armour of my trade: Cap, mask, and gown to prevent blood from splashing onto me and to hide my identity, as any murderer will tell you. I wore gloves to ensure no fingerprints were left behind. Armed with strong steel pliers, I slipped in unnoticed.

I intended to crush his head and end the job quickly, but instinct, perhaps a primitive will to survive, made him turn just then. He backed away. His mouth opened in terror, but the scream never emerged. The steel jaws clamped blindly onto whatever they could grasp.

He twisted and writhed, trying to break free, but my vice-like grip did not relent. Something snapped. I stared in horror at a severed leg in my hand.

The water turned red, splashing everywhere. My victim retreated, but I lunged again. This time, I struck something soft. His abdomen burst open; his guts spilt out. I prided myself on efficiency—yet here I was, creating a gory mess.

Instead of recoiling in horror, I was enraged. How dare he make me feel incompetent? Oblivious to my blood-spattered gown, I chased him like a madman. Finally, I reached the head and crushed the skull. The eyes popped from their sockets, floating on creamy flakes of brain matter carried on a stream of blood.

The job done, I gathered the dismembered limbs, the grotesque torso, the crushed head into a bag. Like a diligent housewife, I scrubbed the area clean. Broken fragments were flushed down the toilet into the sewer. No trace remained, though even my hardened criminal heart wished I had granted a gentler death to one who had never harmed me.

Postscript

This is not a horror story. This is how, with full legal and social sanction, gynaecologists abort an eleven-to-thirteen-week-old foetus. Even a hired assassin would hesitate to murder his victim in such a brutal manner—inserting an instrument blindly in the uterine cavity; now pulling on a leg; now a tiny, perfectly formed, transparent, blue-veined hand; spilling worm-like intestines; not resting until the skull is crushed and dragged through the narrow cervical opening. Like papaya seeds, the eyes float on soft, creamy, squashed brain matter, floating on a thin stream of blood into the bucket.

In earlier times, a laminaria tent (dried seaweed) was inserted into the cervix the night before. It absorbed moisture, gradually dilating the cervix to allow larger instruments to remove the pregnancy piecemeal. Today, a tablet placed vaginally three to four hours earlier achieves the same effect faster and more efficiently.

Despite decades of experience, I still shudder when required to perform a medical termination at this stage.

I hope these graphic details hit hard, because I desperately want people to plan their families before conception—not after—so that pregnancies are prevented, not destroyed. And why should the doctor alone bear the emotional trauma of erasing the by-products of careless pleasure? Perhaps it disturbs them, too, but never enough to stop couples from returning again and again for the same.

27

Unwanted Pregnancies: The Girl Child

On the one hand, I feel compelled to write about that which is a source of shame and sorrow to me as an Indian; on the other, I cannot believe that a day has come when I would call a female child an unwanted by-product of sex. In a country that worships female deities, the girl child—the sweetest creation of God—is being killed indiscriminately, as she has been since time immemorial.

That she would grow up to carry forward the human race, as both procreator and nurturer of mankind, does not deter her killers. That in modern times it is often the rejected one who looks after ageing parents when the son they so hankered for abandons them seems not to matter. She was not wanted centuries ago, and she is not wanted now—period.

Earlier, they drowned her in milk, buried her alive, or stuffed sand into her tiny nostrils and mouth to snuff out her life. Even today, women in Salem, a district in Tamil Nadu, feed the poisonous milk of the *Calotropis* (aak) plant to their newborn daughters and stoically watch them die. It is simply something a woman is expected to do until she proves her worth as the mother of a male child.

My mother once told me the story of a woman on her deathbed, flailing her arms and legs, trying to ward off the demons of her past as they crawled over her flesh to torment her—the eight daughters she had killed in infancy. She begged them to let her die in peace, but it was not to be.

Recently, I made the acquaintance of a woman in her sixties from a rich and respected business family who had a milder form of cerebral palsy. Though her intellect was intact, her speech was slurred and her gait impaired. She told me that even in these modern times, she had nearly been 'bathed' (drowned) in milk for being a second daughter—the cerebral palsy was discovered much later. Her maternal grandmother saved her in the nick of time. Today, she lives an independent, full, and fruitful life, teaching the mentally and physically challenged, and has had numerous partners.

All that advanced technology has accomplished is the early detection and destruction of the female foetus. Sex determination through ultrasound makes it possible to eliminate her in the womb; one no longer has to wait for the birth of a girl child to engineer her death. This discrimination cuts across all strata of society, all castes, and creeds. Neither the rich nor the poor want her. The rich want male heirs to inherit their wealth; the poor must borrow from unscrupulous moneylenders to provide her dowry if she is not raped before marriage. It is the mindset of our people that needs to be changed, not the sex of the child; the practice of dowry that needs to be eliminated, not the girl child.

Despite laws to the contrary, ultrasound-based sex determination continues unabated. Lax enforcement allows such malpractices to flourish; it is a matter of demand and supply, pure and simple. All that has changed is the price, which has risen exponentially now that the practice is clandestine. Even the wily poor, who plead for discounts from compassionate doctors for legitimate treatment, are willing to pay whatever it takes to these specialists. Ingenious methods are used to convey the sex of the foetus—pictures of Ganesh or Lakshmi—since written reports might incriminate the doctor. Occasionally, when the media highlights the skewed sex ratio, a decoy customer is sent, a doctor penalised, and a clinic shut down. More often than not, inspectors are open to bribes. I have heard of one who allegedly took fifty lakh rupees to let a doctor off the hook. It becomes a win–win situation for both law enforcer and lawbreaker. As a result, female foeticide remains very much alive.

To avoid legal hassles, those who can afford it travel to Thailand or similar countries for IVF, even when they can conceive naturally, solely to ensure that only male embryos are transferred to the uterus. Although Indian law prohibits IVF for sex selection in couples with 'secondary infertility' who already have a daughter, selective transfer of male embryos has begun even here.

From the moment of conception, the female child is disadvantaged, at least in India. If she is 'allowed' to live, there are deliberate lapses in her nurturing. She is deprived of adequate nutrition, education, and healthcare, leading to stunted mental and physical development. While her brother is loved and pampered, her body is starved, her mind denied opportunity, and her psyche battered by hostility towards her very existence. Despite this, most girls reach adolescence, for biologically, the female is the stronger sex. She toils from dawn to dusk while her brother goes to school and lords over her like a king. Then there is her vagina—a liability her father must transfer to a husband as soon as he can scrape together the dowry. Meanwhile, her burgeoning sexuality makes her vulnerable to sexual violence. The very men who lament her existence now proceed to violate her—family members, neighbours, acquaintances, strangers. She is spared by none, whether in villages, urban slums, or elite society.

There is a village in one of the northern states where no *baraat* has arrived in decades simply because there are no daughters left to marry. Having mercilessly killed their own, the tall, fair Punjabi race is now importing brides from elsewhere. From a Hitlerian perspective, this may be 'racial dilution', but it is the grim truth.

In some regions a barter system has emerged: A girl is given in marriage only to a family that has a daughter for her brother to marry. One might imagine that the skewed sex ratio would improve the lot of Indian women, that they could choose whom to marry, or whether to marry at all. Sadly, the opposite has occurred. In certain villages, five brothers marry a single woman. Creating the modern-day Draupadi, condemned to a life of endless childbearing and child-rearing.

Where will this end, and how? Why do right-thinking people wallow in apathy? Do they not realise that 'evil prospers when good men do nothing'?

PS Another by-product of irresponsible sexual behaviour is the illegitimate child, a child who suffers physically and mentally throughout life through no fault of their own. Illegitimacy is the only situation in which a male child is meted out the same horrific treatment as a female: Rejection and humiliation. One may ask why, in this era of contraceptives and abortion, anyone would give birth to an illegitimate child. The reasons could be many.

A terrified teenager may hide her head in the sand like an ostrich, as if by ignoring the pregnancy she could wish it away. It could be the result of rape; thinking that it is somehow her fault, the poor girl does not tell anyone. Most unmarried girls are abandoned by their boyfriends at this crucial juncture. Though legally they can seek an MTP after the age of eighteen, doctors insist that a relative accompany them, in case complications occur. They dare not confide in their parents for fear of being thrown out . . . or worse, killed.

Some young girls do not even know that missed periods could mean pregnancy; others have irregular or delayed periods and learn of the pregnancy when it is too late to abort. Yet others have religious restrictions against 'taking life', though premarital sex is also considered a sin in those religions. Whatever the reason, orphanages are full of children nobody wants; the shame of raising a 'bastard' overrides a woman's maternal instincts. Even Kunti placed her illegitimate firstborn, Karna, in a basket and set him afloat on a river.

That a baby can be a source of joy to one and a shame to another never ceases to amaze. One is thrown into a garbage bin; the other is held close to the heart. One is pampered, cocooned in the love of a family, while the other is subjected to a life of humiliation and ostracism. Bruised and battered, deprived of nourishment and education, abused by a society that punishes them for no fault of their own, and propelled towards lives of rebellion and crime, they often end up in delinquent homes.

If only every child were brought into this world because they were wanted; if only people adopted contraceptive measures, adopted these children, or aborted illegitimate pregnancies, the world would be a better place to live in. Alas, it is not so.

I end with a parody of the following poem by Benjamin Franklin:

For want of a nail the shoe was lost.
For want of a shoe the horse was lost.
For want of a horse the rider was lost.
For want of a rider the message was lost.
For want of a message the battle was lost.
For want of a battle the kingdom was lost.
And all for the want of a horseshoe nail.

For want of a condom, she conceived a child.
For want of an abortion, it grew in her womb.
For want of a husband, she delivered a bastard.
For want of a father, he was shamed and abused
And punished, for sins he did not commit
All, for the want of a timely contraceptive.

Acknowledgements

I am indebted to Mr Ashok Chopra for remembering a conversation with an unknown author, over ten years ago. At the conclusion of the Khushwant Singh Lit Fest in Kasauli, he expressed regret at rejecting my book, a rather bold revelation of my interaction with Khushwant Singh, which another publisher accepted soon after. I offered him a book on female sexuality that I was planning to write someday. As a gynaecologist, I was privy to feminine issues that made me realise that a book on women's needs in bed was very much in order. He expressed interest, but no promises were made. Many years and books later, I did come up with such a manuscript, which he accepted graciously.

I cannot thank Sonali Pawar enough for being the editor authors dream of; for going over my manuscript with a fine-toothed comb to bring it to its present readable state.

My heartfelt thanks to Pavan K. Varma, whose modern adaptation of the *Kama Sutra*, *Kama Sutra: The Art of Making Love to a Woman*, was a source of inspiration for my chapter on the subject.

Thanks to Arvind and Shanti Kale for enlightening me on Tantric sexual practices through their book *Tantra: The Secret Power of Sex*.

I am grateful to Satjit Singh for introducing me to the works of the poetess Forugh Farrokhzad, who extolled female sexuality in the conservative Iran of the fifties and paid a heavy price for it.

To Jhumri, my little Shih Tzu, who doesn't know what a comfort her company was during the solitary business of writing.

Last but not least, I would like to express my gratitude to my patients for the insights they gave me on this delicate subject. A kind word and an attentive ear were all it took for their stories to emerge alongside their tears. Many a physical ailment could be traced to a dissatisfaction in their sex life, which urged me to amplify my effort in writing a book that addressed women's needs in bed. Their confessions, like seeds scattered on fertile soil, germinated into stories that I have incorporated into this work.

References

1. Runels, Charles, MD. 2024. 'The Sexual Revolution Has Been Great—For Men.' *MDedge*, 26 September 2024.
2. Jha, Mridulika. 'Hyderabad's Dark Underbelly: Shady "Sheikh Marriages".' *India Today*, 7 Dec. 2024. https://www.indiatoday.in/india/story/hyderabad-mutah-marriages-sheikhs-gulf-countries-minor-girls-investigation-2644868-2024-12-04.
3. Danielsson, Maria, Christina Rogala, and Kajsa Sundström. 'Few Teenage Pregnancies in Sweden—A Comparison Between Five Western Industrialised Countries: Support from and Attitudes in Society Explain the Differences.' *Lakartidningen* 100, no. 30–31 (2003): 2606–2611.
4. Uloko, Maria, Erika P. Isabey, and Blair R. Peters. 2023. 'How Many Nerve Fibers Innervate the Human Glans Clitoris: A Histomorphometric Evaluation of the Dorsal Nerve of the Clitoris.' *The Journal of Sexual Medicine* 20, no. 3 (30 January 2023): 247–52. https://doi.org/10.1093/jsxmed/qdac027.
5. Lemnius, *De occultis naturae miraculis* (1557; English translation *The Secret Miracles of Nature*, London, 1658), cited in Thomas Laqueur, *Making Sex: The Body and Gender from the Greeks to Freud* (Harvard University Press, 1990).
6. Nechay, A., L. M. Ross, J. B. P. Stephenson, and M. O'Regan. 'Gratification Disorder ("Infantile Masturbation"): A Review.' *Archives of Disease in Childhood* 89, no. 3 (March 2004): 225–226. https://doi.org/10.1136/adc.2003.032102.
7. Leiblum, S. R., & Rosen, R. C. (2000). *Principles and Practice of Sex Therapy* (3rd ed.). New York: Guilford Press.
8. Singer, M. I., & McDowall, D. (1988). 'Criminal sexual behaviour in prisons.' *Archives of Sexual Behavior*, 17(3), 261–271.

9. World Health Organization. (2010). *WHO Laboratory Manual for the Examination and Processing of Human Semen* (5th ed.). Geneva: WHO.
10. Kramer, Samuel Noah. *Sumerian Mythology: A Study of Spiritual and Literary Achievement in the Third Millennium BC*. Philadelphia: University of Pennsylvania Press, 1961.
11. Assmann, Jan. *The Mind of Egypt: History and Meaning in the Time of the Pharaohs*. Cambridge, MA: Harvard University Press, 2003.
12. Bailey, J. Michael, Paul L. Vasey, Lisa M. Diamond, S. Marc Breedlove, Eric Vilain, and Marc Epprecht. 'Sexual Orientation, Controversy, and Science.' *Psychological Science in the Public Interest* 17, no. 2 (September 2016): 45–101. https://doi.org/10.1177/1529100616637616.
13. Knight, Daniel A., and Diane Jarrett. 'Preventive Health Care for Women Who Have Sex with Women.' *American Family Physician* 95, no. 5 (1 March 2017): 314–21.
14. Jack Cagney et al., 'Prevalence of Sexual Violence Against Children and Age at First Exposure: A Global Analysis by Location, Age, and Sex (1990–2023),' *The Lancet* 405, no. 10492 (2025): 1817–36, https://doi.org/10.1016/S0140-6736(25)00311-3.
15. Threatened abortion is vaginal bleeding during early pregnancy (usually before 20 weeks) when the cervix remains closed and the pregnancy is still viable.
16. Raymonda Rosen et al., 'The Female Sexual Function Index (FSFI): A Multidimensional Self-Report Instrument for the Assessment of Female Sexual Function,' *Journal of Sex & Marital Therapy* 26, no. 2 (2000): 191–208.
17. Dedden S. J., Werner M. A., Steinweg J, Lissenberg-Witte B. I., Huirne J. A. F., Geomini P. M. A. J., Maas J. W. M. 'Hysterectomy and sexual function: a systematic review and meta-analysis.' *The Journal of Sexual Medicine*. 2023;20(4):447–466. DOI: 10.1093/jsxmed/qdac051.

'The gateways to wisdom and knowledge are always open.'

Louise Hay